Clinical Ethics

A Practical Approach to Ethical Decisions in Clinical Medicine

Seventh Edition

Albert R. Jonsen, PhD
Professor Emeritus of Ethics in Medicine
University of Washington School of Medicine
Seattle, Washington
Senior Ethics Scholar in Residence
California Pacific Medical Center
San Francisco, California

Mark Siegler, MD
Lindy Bergman Distinguished Service Professor of Medicine and Surgery
Director, MacLean Center for Clinical Medical Ethics
University of Chicago
Chicago, Illinois

William J. Winslade, PhD, JD
James Wade Rockwell Professor of Philosophy in Medicine
Institute for the Medical Humanities
Professor of Psychiatry and Preventive Medicine and Community Health
University of Texas Medical Branch
Galveston, Texas

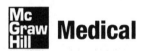 **Medical**

New York Chicago San Francisco Lisbon London Madrid Mexico City
Milan New Delhi San Juan Seoul Singapore Sydney Toronto

Clinical Ethics: A Practical Approach to Ethical Decisions in Clinical Medicine, Seventh Edition

1 2 3 4 5 6 7 8 9 0 DOC/DOC 14 13 12 11 10

ISBN 978-0-07-163414-4
MHID 0-07-163414-2

This book was set in Times and Garamond by Aptara Inc.
The editors were James Shanahan and Christine Diedrich.
The production supervisor was Catherine Saggese.
Project management was provided by Samir Roy, Aptara Inc.
The cover designer was Mary McKeon
RR Donnelley was the printer and binder.

This book is printed on acid-free paper.   1006284151

Library of Congress Cataloging-in-Publication Data

Jonsen, Albert R.
    Clinical ethics : a practical approach to ethical decisions in clinical medicine / Albert R. Jonsen, Mark Siegler, William J. Winslade. —7th ed.
        p. ; cm.
    Includes bibliographical references and index.
    Summary: "This book is about the ethical issues that clinicians encounter in caring for patients. In order to practice excellent clinical care, clinicians and those studying to become clinicians must understand ethical issues such as informed consent, truth telling, confidentiality, privacy, the distinction between research and clinical care, and end-of-life care. Our audience also includes families and other persons close to patients, who may participate in decisions about their care"—Provided by publisher.
    ISBN-13: 978-0-07-163414-4 (alk. paper)
    ISBN-10: 0-07-163414-2 (alk. paper)
    1. Medical ethics.   2. Medical ethics—Case studies.   I. Siegler, Mark, 1941–
II. Winslade, William J.   III. Title.
    [DNLM: 1. Ethics, Clinical.   2. Bioethical Issues.   3. Decision Making.   4. Ethical Analysis—methods.   5. Patient Participation.   6. Quality of Life.
    WB 60 J81c 2010]
    R724.J66 2010
    174.2—dc22
                                                    2010001195

McGraw-Hill books are available at special quantity discounts to use as premiums and sales promotions, or for use in corporate training programs. To contact a representative, please e-mail us at bulksales@mcgraw-hill.com.

WITHD 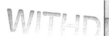 **Clinical Ethics**

DATE DUE FOR RETURN

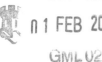
This book may be recalled before the above date.

Contents

Introduction

This book is about the ethical issues that clinicians encounter in caring for patients. In order to practice excellent clinical care, clinicians and those studying to become clinicians must understand ethical issues such as informed consent, truth telling, confidentiality, privacy, the distinction between research and clinical care, and end-of-life care. Clinicians must apply this knowledge in their daily practices. By clinicians we mean not only physicians and surgeons but also nurses, social workers, psychologists, clinical ethicists, medical technicians, chaplains, and others responsible for the welfare of patients. Some of these clinicians will also be members of ethics committees who deliberate about the ethics policies of their hospitals and about ethical problems in particular cases. Our audience also includes families and other persons close to patients, who may participate in decisions about their care. Our goal in writing this book is to help clinicians understand and manage the cases they encounter in their practices, and on those occasions when ethical disagreements emerge, to guide patients, families, clinicians, and ethics committees toward the resolution of clinical ethical conflicts.

Ethical issues are imbedded in every clinical encounter between patients and caregivers because the care of patients always involves both technical and moral considerations. The central feature of this clinical encounter is the therapeutic relationship between a physician and a patient, a relationship that is permeated with ethical responsibilities. Physicians must aim, in the words of Hippocrates, "to help and do no harm." Modern physicians approach the doctor–patient relationship with a professional identity that includes the obligations to provide competent care to the patient, to preserve confidentiality, and to communicate honestly and compassionately.

In the usual course of a therapeutic relationship, clinical care and ethical duties run smoothly together. The reason is that generally the patient and physician share the same goal: to respond to the medical problems and needs of the patient. For example, a patient presents with a distressing cough and wants relief; a physician responds to the patient by utilizing the correct means to diagnose and treat this condition. In this situation, the treatment for, say, a mild asthma attack is effective and the patient is satisfied. At the same time an ethical action has taken place: the patient is helped and not harmed. In other cases, this simple scene becomes complicated. The patient's asthma may be caused by a cancer obstructing the airway. This disease may be life-threatening and the treatment may be complex, difficult and may prove unsuccessful. On other occasions, the smooth course of the doctor–patient relationship may be interrupted by what we call an ethical question: a doubt about the right action when ethical responsibilities conflict or when their meaning is uncertain or confused. For example, the physician's duty to cure is countered by a patient's refusal of indicated treatment, or the patient cannot afford treatment because of lack of insurance. The principles that usually bring the clinician and the patient into a therapeutic relationship seem to collide. This collision blocks the process of deciding and acting that is intrinsic to clinical care. This confusion and conflict can become distressing for all parties. This book, then, aims to elucidate both the ethical dimensions of care in ordinary clinical activities that are not controversial, as well as when doubt about right action blocks decision.

Clinical ethics, then, is a structured approach to ethical questions in clinical medicine. Clinical ethics depends on the larger discipline of bioethics, which in turn draws upon disciplines such as moral philosophy, health law, communication skills, and clinical medicine. The scholars called "bioethicists" must master this field. However, clinicians in the daily practice of medicine can manage with a basic understanding of certain key ethical issues such as informed consent and end-of-life care. *Central to the practical application of clinical ethics is the ability to identify and analyze an ethical question and to reach a reasonable conclusion and recommendation for action.* In this book, we provide a method to identify the ethical dimensions of patient care and to analyze and resolve ethical problems. This method is useful for structuring the questions faced by any clinician who cares for patients.

THE FOUR TOPICS

Bioethics identifies four ethical principles that are particularly relevant to clinical medicine: the principles of beneficence, nonmaleficence, respect for autonomy, and justice. To these, some bioethicists add empathy, compassion, fidelity, integrity, and other virtues. The bioethical literature discusses these principles and virtues at length. In this book, we only explain them briefly. We rather direct our reader's attention to how these general principles interact within the concrete circumstances of a clinical case, and how they serve as guides to action in specific circumstances. Thus we propose four topics that we believe constitute the essential structure of a case in clinical medicine, namely, medical indications, patient preferences, quality of life, and contextual features.

Some users of this book call these four topics "the Four Boxes." Every clinical case is a mass of detail that the clinician must interpret in order to carry out the reasoning process necessary for diagnosis and treatment. Every clinician learns early in training a common pattern for organizing that mass of detail: chief complaint, history of the chief complaint, general medical history of the patient, results of physical examination, and results of laboratory studies. The data that are sorted into these patterns lead the clinician to decisions about diagnosis and treatment. Our four topics or boxes provide a similar pattern for collecting, sorting, and ordering the facts of a clinical *ethical* problem. Each topic or "box" is filled with the actual facts of the clinical case that are relevant to the identification of the ethical problem, and the contents of all four are viewed together for a comprehensive picture of the ethical dimensions of the case.

Medical indications refer to the diagnostic and therapeutic interventions that are being used to evaluate and treat the medical problem in the case. Patient preferences state the express choices of the patient about their treatment, or the decisions of those who are authorized to speak for the patient when the patient is incapable of doing so. Quality of life describes features of the patient's life prior to and following treatment, insofar as these features are pertinent to medical decisions. Contextual features identify the familial, social, institutional, financial, and legal settings within which the particular case takes place, insofar as they influence medical decisions. Under each of these headings, a series of questions are posed to assure that needed information has been gathered. We believe that these four topics are the essential and constant constituents of any clinical case, which is, of course, unique and varying in its own circumstances. The chart at the end of this introduction depicts these four topics and the relevant questions.

The subtitle of our book states that clinical ethics is a *practical* approach. This implies that the approach must go beyond simply identifying the problem, by collecting and sorting the facts of the case. It must guide practice, that is, it must lead from identification of the ethical problem to decisions about how to manage the problem. It must show the clinician how to manage those obstacles to decision making that the ethical problem had posed. Clinical ethics is seldom a matter of deciding between ethical versus unethical, between good and right versus bad and wrong; rather it involves finding the better, most reasonable solutions among the relevant options. While clinical ethics can sometimes help to rule out options that are unethical, more frequently, clinical ethics can clarify a range of permissible options that patients and clinicians may choose. Our approach seeks to guide the clinician, and others involved in the case, toward such resolutions.

After all relevant information is gathered into the Four Boxes, the relationship between that information and the principles must be assessed. It sometimes happens that when the data is collected and properly sorted, an obvious pattern appears that will identify the ethical problem. The circumstances of a case often point to one of the fundamental principles as most important in the specific case analysis. For example, a patient has a critical disease in its terminal stage, has never expressed preferences about treatment, has no relatives to speak for him, and faces great suffering during the time remaining. This appears at first sight as a case in which the principles of beneficence and nonmaleficence are central. Further, aggressive treatment is no longer likely to be beneficial; this patient needs palliative care. At second sight, however, the question becomes a matter of the principle of respect for autonomy: who is authorized to make the decision to transition from intensive to palliative care? Ethical reflection moves from this dilemma between two fundamental principles to an evaluation of how the circumstances of the case give greater weight to one or the other of these principles. For example, after all reasonable attempts to effectively treat a patient have failed, the continued application of aggressive measures causes more harm than good to this patient. In this light, the principle of nonmaleficence becomes the most dominant one, and provides an ethical reason for a decision to provide only palliative care. The clinician can then formulate a recommendation to the patient or other decision makers.

This resolution of the case is based on an assessment of the facts of the case in relation to the ethical principles relevant to the case. However, this assessment calls for a further move: the present case must be compared to similar cases. It is certainly true that in medicine every case is unique, and every patient "a statistic of one." Nevertheless, the case at hand will have similarities with other cases. Other cases may have been thoughtfully considered—perhaps even adjudicated in the law—and may provide guidance whereby to assess the present case. *Such cases are called paradigm cases.* Reference to paradigm cases do not prove that a case is correctly assessed; rather they are examples of serious assessments in prior, similar cases, to which the current case can be compared, in order to guide the clinician in this case. It is important to note that even similar cases have variable nuances. The present case may have circumstances that make it more complex than previous cases; or it may represent a novel problem due to innovative technology. Clinicians and ethicists should be familiar with these paradigm cases, and be able to discern how they differ and how the circumstances bond with principles in the current case. We describe some of the important paradigm cases.

This book is arranged to follow the four-box model. Each chapter is devoted to one of the four topics. Each chapter begins with some general considerations and ethical principles most relevant to that topic. A series of questions that exemplify major issues under each topic are posed. Clinical situations that commonly generate ethical problems associated with that topic are stated and illustrated by cases. A COMMENT that provides a distillation of prevailing opinion from the bioethical literature follows. We conclude with RECOMMENDATIONS that the three authors formulate from their own extensive experience as clinicians and clinical ethics consultants. Although this book does not discuss pediatric ethics, at the end of each chapter we have placed "Pediatric Notes" to alert readers about certain ethical problems in pediatric medicine that require special consideration. When these arise, the sources for pediatric ethics should be consulted. One such source is Frankel LR, Goldworth A, Rorty MV, Silverman WD. *Ethical Dilemmas in Pediatrics.* Cambridge, MA: Cambridge University Press; 2005.

RESOURCES IN CLINICAL ETHICS

In addition to our method for identifying and assessing a case in ethical terms, we also provide capsules of essential information about common problems, such as Orders Not to Resuscitate or Withholding Life Support. The issues that we treat in capsule form have been discussed and debated in the ever-increasing literature of bioethics. We refer readers to certain sources where they can find more extended discussions and references, and complete references are provided at the end of this section. The standard text of scholarly bioethics, in which basic concepts are amply explained, is *Principles of Biomedical Ethics.* The major reference work in medical ethics is *Encyclopedia of Bioethics*. We regularly refer to three books that contain fuller treatments of the matters that we treat only in capsule form. They are *Resolving Ethical Dilemmas: A Guide for Clinicians*; *The Oxford Handbook of Bioethics*; and *The Cambridge Textbook of Bioethics*. Our pages regularly refer to their relevant chapters. Another book collects cases that represent difficult problems confronting clinical ethicists: *Complex Ethics Consultations: Cases that Haunt Us*. A number of journals are now dedicated to bioethics: *The Hastings Center Report, The American Journal of Bioethics, Journal of Medical Ethics, Cambridge Quarterly of Healthcare Ethics, Journal of Theoretical Medicine,* and *Journal of Clinical Ethics.* Also, articles on bioethics appear regularly in the medical and nursing journals. We do not reference this extensive journal literature, unless we use data drawn from an article or an article is "classic" in defining and describing an issue. This literature is indexed at PubMed and Medline at the National Library of Medicine's Bioethics Portal (www.nlm.nih.gov/bsd/bioethics.html). Extensive bibliographic resources can be found at the National Reference Center for Bioethics Literature at Georgetown University's ETHXWeb (http://bioethics.georgetown.edu/databases/index.htm); Clinical Ethics Center of the National Institutes of Health (www.nih.gov/sigs/bioethics); and, for cases and discussions, the American Medical Association's online journal Virtual Mentor is an excellent resource (http://virtualmentor.ama-assn.org). The Web site UpToDate (www.uptodate.com) contains a number of useful reviews of major topics, as does the Web site of the University of Washington Department of Bioethics and Humanities (http://depts.washington.edu/bhdept). Of less relevance to ethics at the bedside, but still helpful, is United Nations Educational, Scientific and Cultural Organization's Global Ethics Observatory (http://www.unesco.org/shs/ethics/geobs). Also see McGraw-Hill's AccessMedicine Web site (www.accessmedicine.com) for thousands of images and illustrations, interactive assessment, case files, diagnostic tools, and up-to-date information for research, education, self-assessment, and board review.

ACKNOWLEDGEMENTS

The authors gratefully acknowledge the advice and assistance of the following people: Drs. Katrina Bramstedt, David Brush, Michael Cantwell, Farr Curlin, Lainie Ross, William Stewart, and Daniel Sulmasy, as well as Ms. Helene Starks, Ms. Donna Vickers, and Mr. Wesley McGaughey.

BIBLIOGRAPHY

American Journal of Bioethics. Taylor and Francis Group Inc. http://www. bioethics.net.

Beauchamp TL, Childress JF. *Principles of Biomedical Ethics*. 6th ed. New York, NY: Oxford University Press; 2009.

Cambridge Quarterly of Healthcare Ethics. 40 West 20th Street, New York, NY 10011–4211. http://www.journals.cup.org.

Ford PJ, Dudzinski DM. *Complex Ethics Consultations: Cases that Haunt Us*. New York, NY: Cambridge University Press; 2008

Frankel LR, Goldworth A, Rorty MV, Silverman WA, eds. *Ethical Dilemmas in Pediatrics*. New York, NY: Cambridge University Press; 2005.

Journal of Clinical Ethics. 17100 Cole Road, Hagerstown, MD 21740. http://www.clinicalethics.com.

Journal of Medical Ethics. BMJ Publishing Group, British Medical Association, Tavistock Square London WCIH 9JR, UK. http://www.jme.bmj.com.

Lo B. *Resolving Ethical Dilemmas: A Guide for Clinicians*. 4th ed. Philadelphia, PA: Lippincott Williams & Wilkins; 2009.

Post SG, ed. *Encyclopedia of Bioethics*. 3rd ed. Farmington Hills, MI: Gale; 2003.

Singer PA, Viens AM. *The Cambridge Textbook of Bioethics*. New York, NY: Cambridge University Press; 2008.

Steinbock B, ed. *The Oxford Handbook of Bioethics*. New York, NY: Oxford University Press; 2009.

The Hastings Center Report. The Hastings Center, Garrison, NY, 10524–5555. E-mail: mail@thehastingscenter.org; http://www.thehastingscenter.org.

Walters L, Kahn TJ, eds. *Bibliography of Bioethics*. Washington, DC: Georgetown University Press. [Published annually].

The Four Topics Chart

Medical Indications	Patient References
The Principles of Beneficence and Nonmaleficence 1. What is the patient's medical problem? Is the problem acute? chronic? critical? reversible? emergent? terminal? 2. What are the goals of treatment? 3. In what circumstances are medical treatments not indicated? 4. What are the probabilities of success of various treatment options? 5. In sum, how can this patient be benefited by medical and nursing care, and how can harm be avoided?	The Principle of Respect for Autonomy 1. Has the patient been informed of benefits and risks, understood this information, and given consent? 2. Is the patient mentally capable and legally competent, and is there evidence of incapacity? 3. If mentally capable, what preferences about treatment is the patient stating? 4. If incapacitated, has the patient expressed prior preferences? 5. Who is the appropriate surrogate to make decisions for the incapacitated patient? 6. Is the patient unwilling or unable to cooperate with medical treatment? If so, why?

Quality of Life	Contextual Features
The Principles of Beneficence and Nonmaleficence and Respect for Autonomy 1. What are the prospects, with or without treatment, for a return to normal life, and what physical, mental, and social deficits might the patient experience even if treatment succeeds? 2. On what grounds can anyone judge that some quality of life would be undesirable for a patient who cannot make or express such a judgment? 3. Are there biases that might prejudice the provider's evaluation of the patient's quality of life? 4. What ethical issues arise concerning improving or enhancing a patient's quality of life? 5. Do quality-of-life assessments raise any questions regarding changes in treatment plans, such as forgoing life-sustaining treatment? 6. What are plans and rationale to forgo life-sustaining treatment? 7. What is the legal and ethical status of suicide?	The Principles of Justice and Fairness 1. Are there professional, interprofessional, or business interests that might create conflicts of interest in the clinical treatment of patients? 2. Are there parties other than clinicians and patients, such as family members, who have an interest in clinical decisions? 3. What are the limits imposed on patient confidentiality by the legitimate interests of third parties? 4. Are there financial factors that create conflicts of interest in clinical decisions? 5. Are there problems of allocation of scarce health resources that might affect clinical decisions? 6. Are there religious issues that might influence clinical decisions? 7. What are the legal issues that might affect clinical decisions? 8. Are there considerations of clinical research and education that might affect clinical decisions? 9. Are there issues of public health and safety that affect clinical decisions? 10. Are there conflicts of interest within institutions and organizations (e.g., hospitals) that may affect clinical decisions and patient welfare?

Medical Indications

T his chapter treats the first topic relevant to any ethical problem in clinical medicine, namely, the indications for or against medical intervention. In most cases, treatment decisions that are based on medical indications are straightforward and present no obvious ethical problems.

EXAMPLE. A patient complains of frequent urination accompanied by a burning sensation. The physician suspects a urinary tract infection, obtains a confirmatory culture, and prescribes an antibiotic. The physician explains to the patient the nature of the condition and the reason for prescribing the medication. The patient obtains the prescription, takes the medication, and is cured of the infection.

This is a case of clinical ethics, not because it shows an *ethical problem*, but because it demonstrates how the principles commonly considered necessary for ethical medical care, namely, respect for autonomy, beneficence, nonmaleficence, and justice, are satisfied in the clinical circumstances of this case. Medical indications are sufficiently clear so that the physician can make a diagnosis and prescribe an effective therapy to benefit the patient. The patient's preferences coincide with the physician's recommendations. The patient's quality of life, presently made unpleasant by the infection, is improved. This case occurs in a context in which medications are available, insurance pays the bill, and no problems with family or institution are present.

This case, which raises no ethical concerns, would present an ethical problem if the patient stated that he did not believe in antibiotics, or if the urinary tract infection developed in the last days of a terminal illness, or if the infection was associated with a sexually transmitted disease in which sexual partners might be endangered, or if the patient could not pay for the care. Sometimes, these problems can be readily resolved; at other times, they can become major obstacles in the management of the case.

In this chapter, we first define medical indications and explain the ethical principles most relevant to medical indications, namely, beneficence and nonmaleficence. We discuss the relationship of these principles to medical professionalism. We then pose a series of questions that link medical indications to these principles. In discussing these questions, we treat important features of clinical medicine related to medical indications, including the goals and benefits of medicine, clinical judgment and uncertainty, evidence-based medicine, and medical error. We offer typical cases to illustrate these discussions. We then consider three ethical issues in which medical indications are particularly prominent: (1) nonbeneficial (or futile) treatment, (2) cardiopulmonary resuscitation (CPR) and do-not-resuscitate (DNR) orders, and (3) the determination of death.

1.0.1 Definition of Medical Indications

Medical Indications are the facts, opinions, and interpretations about the patient's physical and/or psychological condition that provide a reasonable basis for diagnostic and therapeutic activities aiming to realize the overall goals of medicine: prevention, cure, and care of illness and injury. Every discussion of an ethical problem in clinical medicine should begin with a statement of medical indications. In the usual clinical presentation, this review of indications for medical intervention leads to the determination of goals and the formulation of recommendations to the patient. *Therefore, medical indications are those facts about the patient's physiological or psychological condition that indicate which forms of diagnostic, therapeutic, or educational interventions are appropriate.*

1.0.2 The Ethical Principles of Beneficence and Nonmaleficence

Medical Indications describe the day-to-day work of clinical care for patients—diagnosing their condition and providing helpful treatments. The ethical principles that should govern these activities are the principles of beneficence and nonmaleficence, that is, acting so as to benefit the patients and not harm them. The most ancient moral maxim of medicine, stated in the Hippocratic oath, is "I will use treatment to benefit the sick according to my ability and judgment but never with a view to injury and wrongdoing." Another Hippocratic imperative to physicians states, "be of benefit and do no harm" (*Epidemics I*). There are many ways to benefit persons, for example, by educating, hiring, and promoting an employee; giving a recommendation; and making a gift. There are also many ways to harm, for example, by slandering, stealing, and beating. In medicine, benefit and harm have a specific meaning: helping by trying to heal and doing so as safely and painlessly as possible.

Therefore, in medical ethics, *beneficence primarily means the duty to try to bring about those improvements in physical or psychological health that medicine can achieve.* These objective effects of diagnostic and therapeutic actions are, for example, diagnosing and curing an infection, treating cancer that leads to remission, and facilitating the healing of a fracture. *Nonmaleficence means going about these activities in ways that prevent further injury or reduce its risk.* So, this topic will treat medical benefits as objective contributions to the health of a patient. The subjective aspects of patients' choices, that is, their estimate of the value and utility that medical contributions bring to them personally and their acceptance and rejection of them, are discussed under Topic Two, "Patient Preferences," and Topic Three, "Quality of Life."

Beauchamp TL, Childress JF. Chapter 4: Nonmaleficence; Chapter 5: Beneficence. In: Beauchamp TL, Childress JF, eds. *Principles of Biomedical Ethics.* 6th ed. New York, NY: Oxford University Press; 2009:140–186; 197–239.

1.0.3 Benefit–Risk Ratio

In medicine, beneficence and nonmaleficence are assessed in what is called "Benefit–Risk Ratio" reasoning. It would be clearly wrong for a physician to set out to harm a patient, but it is almost inevitable that when a physician attempts to benefit a patient, by medication or surgery, for example, some harm or risk of harm is possible or may ensue. Every surgical procedure causes a wound; most drugs have adverse effects. Therefore, the principles of beneficence and nonmaleficence do not merely instruct the clinician to help and do no harm; they coalesce to guide the clinician's assessment of how much risk is justified by the intended benefit. A physician must calculate this "ratio" and fashion it into a recommendation to the patient who will, in the last analysis, evaluate it in light of his or her own values.

Examples. (1) A patient with asthma and diabetes needs a course of steroids for worsening asthma, but the doctor knows that steroids will make diabetes control more difficult. (2) A surgeon takes a beta-blocking drug to decrease tremor before operating, but the use of the beta-blocker exacerbates his asthma.

1.0.4 The Therapeutic Relationship and Professionalism

The competence of a physician to benefit the patient by his or her medical knowledge and skill, as well as the expectation and desire of the patient to be benefited by these skills, is a key moral aspect of a therapeutic relationship. The principles of beneficence and nonmaleficence are the central ethical aspects of this relationship. This therapeutic relationship has further implications for physicians as professionals.

As the *Charter on Medical Professionalism* states, professionalism "demands placing the interest of patients above those of the physician, setting and maintaining standards of competence and integrity, and providing expert advice to society on matters of health." Professionalism encourages placing care for the patient ahead of the business of medicine. This implies that physicians should primarily pursue the goals of medicine in their dealings with patients, rather than favoring personal, private goals. More directly, physicians must avoid exploitation of patients for their own profit or reputation. The benefits of medicine are optimal when physicians and other health professionals demonstrate a professionalism that includes honesty and integrity, respect for patients, a commitment to patients' welfare, a compassionate regard for patients, and a dedication to maintain competency in knowledge and technical skills. In manifesting these virtues, professionalism and ethics are linked. The ethical and professional responsibilities of physicians are closely tied to their ability to fulfill the goals of medicine in conjunction with their respect for patients' preferences about the goals of their lives.

Charter on Medical Professionalism. *Ann Intern Med.* 2002;136:243–246; *Lancet.* 2002;359:520–522.
Dugdale LS, Siegler M, Rubin DT. Medical professionalism: crossing a generational divide. *Perspect Biol Med.* 2008;51(4):554–564.

1.0.5 A Clinical Approach to Beneficence and Nonmaleficence

The general principles of beneficence and nonmaleficence must be situated in the clinical circumstances of the patient. In order to do this, we propose that clinicians first consider the topic of Medical Indications. We ask five questions that define the scope of the topic of Medical Indications. These questions form the structure of this chapter. In answering them, we will explain how the clinical circumstances are linked to the principles of beneficence and nonmaleficence. These five questions are as follows:

1. What is the patient's medical problem? Is the problem acute? chronic? critical? reversible? emergent? terminal?
2. What are the goals of treatment?
3. In what circumstances are medical treatments not indicated?
4. What are the probabilities of success of various treatment options?
5. In sum, how can this patient be benefited by medical and nursing care, and how can harm be avoided?

1.0.6 Question One—What Is the Patient's Medical Problem? Is the Problem Acute? Chronic? Critical? Reversible? Emergent? Terminal?

Clinical medicine is not abstract; it deals with particular patients who present with particular health problems. Therefore, clinical ethics must begin with as clear and detailed a picture as possible of those problems. This picture is usually obtained through the standard methods of clinical medicine—history, physical diagnosis, data from laboratory studies—interpreted against a background of clinical experience. This leads to a differential diagnosis, as well as a management plan for further diagnostic tests and for treatment. As clinicians synthesize and organize the patient's case, they consider the issues discussed below in Question 2.

1.0.7 Important Distinctions: Is the Problem Acute? Chronic? Critical? Reversible? Emergent? Terminal?

Any differential diagnosis or treatment option will implicitly answer these questions. However, it is important to raise them explicitly at the time of an ethics discussion or consultation. The ethical implications of particular choices are often significantly influenced by the answer to these questions. Persons involved in an ethics discussion, such as the family of a patient or an ethics committee member, may not be fully aware of these important features. It is necessary to be clear about whether the ethical problem pertains to an acute reversible condition of a patient who has a terminal disease (such as pneumonia in a patient with widely metastatic cancer) or to an acute episode of a chronic condition (such as ketoacidosis in a diabetic patient). Therefore, the following points must be clear to all participants in an ethics discussion:

(a) *The disease*: A disease may be *acute* (rapid onset and short course) or *chronic* (persistent and progressive). It can be an *emergency* (causing immediate disability unless treated) or a *nonemergency* (slowly progressive). Finally, a disease can be *curable* (the primary cause is known and treatable by definitive therapy) or *incurable*.

(b) *The treatment*: Proposed treatments depend on the particular disease being treated. Patients' decisions about treatment will vary on the basis of their goals, desires, and values. A medical intervention may be *burdensome* (known to cause serious adverse effects) or *nonburdensome* (unlikely to have serious side effects). The potential burdens of an intervention are considered by patients and physicians when deciding on a treatment plan. In addition, interventions may be *curative* (offering definitive correction of a condition) or *supportive* (offering relief of symptoms and slowing the progression of diseases that are currently incurable). For certain progressive diseases such as diabetes, supportive intervention, such as tight glycemic control, can be very efficacious, stopping or reversing disease progression and allowing the patient to maintain a high quality of life for many years. For other conditions, such as amyotrophic lateral sclerosis (Lou Gehrig disease) or Alzheimer disease, interventions and treatments rarely delay the progression of disease but may palliate symptoms and successfully treat acute episodes.

1.0.8 Four Typical Cases

We offer four typical patients who will reappear throughout this book as our major examples. The patients in these cases are given the names Mr. Cure, Ms. Cope, Mr. Care, and Ms. Comfort. These pseudonyms are chosen to suggest prominent features of their medical condition. Mr. Cure suffers from bacterial meningitis, a serious but curable acute condition. Ms. Cope has a chronic condition, insulin-dependent diabetes that requires not only continual medical treatment but also the patient's active involvement in her own care. Mr. Care has multiple sclerosis (MS), a disease that cannot currently be cured but whose inexorable deterioration can sometimes be delayed by treatments and always can be alleviated by good medical care. Ms. Comfort has breast cancer that has metastasized, for which there is a low probability of cure even under a regimen of intensive intervention.

CASE I. Mr. Cure, a 24-year-old graduate student, has been brought to the emergency room (ER) by a friend. Previously in good health, he is complaining of a severe headache and stiff neck. Physical examination shows a somnolent patient without focal neurologic signs but with a temperature of 39.5°C and nuchal rigidity. An examination of spinal fluid reveals cloudy fluid with a white blood cell count of 2000; a Gram stain of the fluid shows many gram-positive diplococci. A diagnosis of bacterial meningitis is made; administration of antibiotics is recommended.

COMMENT. In this case, the medical indications are the clinical data that suggest a diagnosis of bacterial meningitis for which a specific therapy, namely, administration of antibiotics, is appropriate. Nothing yet suggests that this case poses any ethical problem. However, in Topic Two, we shall see how ethical problems emerge from what appears to be a noncontroversial clinical situation: Mr. Cure will refuse therapy. That refusal will cause consternation among the physicians and the nurses caring for him; it will also raise an ethical conflict between the duty of physicians to benefit the patient versus the autonomy of the patient. When that problem appears, clinicians may be tempted to leap directly to the ethical problems of the patient's refusal. We suggest that the first step in ethical analysis not be such a leap but rather a clear exposition of the medical indications. Analysis should begin with answers to the questions, "What is the diagnosis?" "What are the medical indications for treatment?" "What are the probabilities of success?" "What are the consequences of failure to treat?" and "Are there any reasonable alternatives for treating this clinical problem?"

CASE II. Ms. Cope is a 42-year-old woman whose insulin-dependent diabetes was diagnosed at age 18. Despite good compliance with an insulin and dietary regimen, she experienced frequent episodes of ketoacidosis and hypoglycemia, which necessitated repeated hospitalizations and ER care. For the last few years, her diabetes has been controlled with an implanted insulin pump. Twenty-four years after the onset of diabetes, she has no functional impairment from her disease. However, fundoscopic examination reveals a moderate number of microaneurysms, and urinalysis shows increased microalbuminuria.

CASE III. Mr. Care, a 44-year-old man, was diagnosed with MS 15 years ago. For the past 12 years, he has experienced progressive deterioration and has not responded to the medications currently approved to delay MS progression. He is now confined to a wheelchair and for 2 years has required an indwelling Foley catheter because of an atonic bladder. In the last year, he has become profoundly depressed, is uncommunicative even with close family, and rarely rises from bed.

CASE IV. Ms. Comfort is a 58-year-old woman with metastatic breast cancer. Three years ago, she underwent a mastectomy with reconstruction. Dissected nodes revealed infiltrative disease. She received several courses of chemotherapy and radiation.

COMMENT. In these four cases, we present a very simplified picture of patients seen in terms of medical indications, that is, diagnosis and treatment. No particular ethical problems are described. As the book advances, various problems will arise that merit the name *clinical ethical problems*. Some of these are related to changes in medical indications themselves, whereas some are due to the patients' preferences, their quality of life, and the context of care. Topics Two, Three, and Four treat these questions. Mr. Cure, Ms. Cope, Mr. Care, and Ms. Comfort will appear frequently in the coming pages. Details of these cases will occasionally be changed to illustrate various points as the text proceeds. In addition to these four model cases, many other case examples will appear in which the patients will be designated by initials.

The first question of Topic One, which examines the patient's immediate presenting problems, as well as the patient's overall clinical condition, is centrally important in developing both a clinical and an ethical analysis of the situation. This information is the sort usually found in the patient's chart. *We emphasize that any clinical assessment or any ethics consultation must begin with a complete review of this information.* We also emphasize that in some cases, an ethics consultation by a clinically knowledgeable ethicist might reveal that some important information is missing and that clinicians should be encouraged to obtain it to make the ethical analysis more relevant and helpful.

1.0.9 Question Two—What Are the Goals of Treatment?

In order to understand the ethical issues in a case, it is necessary to consider the clinical situation of the patient, that is, the nature of the disease, the treatment proposed, and the goals of intervention. The analysis and resolution of an ethical issue often depend on a clear perception of these factors. The general goals of medicine are as follows:

1. Cure of disease
2. Maintenance or improvement of quality of life through relief of symptoms, pain, and suffering

3. Promotion of health and prevention of disease
4. Prevention of untimely death
5. Improvement of functional status or maintenance of compromised status
6. Education and counseling of patients regarding their condition and prognosis
7. Avoidance of harm to the patient in the course of care
8. Providing relief and support near time of death

In every particular case, these general goals are made specific by understanding the nature of the disease(s) involved in the case and the range of available, appropriate treatment. Therefore, attention must be paid to the distinctions stated above (see Section 1.0.7), as specific to the patient's disease and to the particular circumstances of the patient.

In many cases, most of the general goals of medicine can be achieved simultaneously. For example, in the case of Mr. Cure and his bacterial meningitis, a course of antibiotics should cure the disease; relieve the symptoms, such as headache and fever; protect his nervous system from damage; and restore his health (therefore, avoiding the need for support in time of death). However, at times, goals will conflict. For example, when considering the use of antihypertensive drugs, the goal of reducing the risk of heart attack and stroke may conflict with the goal of avoiding harmful side effects, such as impotence and fatigue, that will impair a patient's quality of life. In other cases, goals such as curing disease may be impossible to achieve because of a patient's advanced condition and/or limitations in scientific and medical knowledge. In every medical case, the goals must be clear and conflicts between goals must be understood and managed, as much as possible.

An old medical maxim sums up the goals of medicine concisely: "cure sometimes, relieve often, comfort always." While the old maxim remains true, modern medicine has changed its application. Cure is much more often achieved now than in the past: developments in anesthesia and asepsis have expanded surgical possibilities, and the development of modern pharmacology has expanded effective medical treatments. Many chronic diseases that were once lethal can now be effectively managed. In recent years, the medical profession has taken more seriously the mandate to "comfort always" and has improved its ability to provide palliation to chronically and terminally ill patients.

An ethical problem may appear in a case if the goals of intervention are poorly defined, are unclear or confused, or are overtaken by the rapid course of disease—goals that are perfectly reasonable when a patient is admitted for surgery may no longer be reasonable when, postoperatively, the patient becomes septic. Sometimes the ethical problem merely reflects a failure to clarify for all participants the feasible goals that the physician has identified; at other times, there may be a genuine conflict between goals. Clinical ethics consultation may assist clinicians to clarify when cure is possible, how long intensive medical interventions should be continued, and when comfort should become the primary mode of care.

In every case, patients and physicians should clarify the goals of intervention when deciding on a course of treatment. This clarification entails, first of all, the physician's knowledge and skill in diagnosis and treatment: he or she must, to the extent possible in a given clinical setting, set and reset goals realistically. In addition, he or she must take account of the patient's own goals (Topic Two, "Patient Preferences," and Topic Three, "Quality of Life").

1.1 INDICATED AND NONINDICATED INTERVENTIONS

1.1.1 Question Three: In What Circumstances Are Medical Treatments Not Indicated?

One of the major sources of ethical problems is the determination whether a particular intervention is, or is not, indicated. Innumerable interventions are available to modern medicine, from counseling to drugs to surgery. In any particular clinical case, only some of these available interventions are indicated, that is, only some interventions are clearly related to the needs and data of the clinical situation and to the goals of medicine. The competent clinician always judges what intervention is indicated for the case at hand. *Therefore, the term "medically indicated" describes what a sound clinical judgment determines to be physiologically and medically appropriate in the circumstances of a particular case.*

Interventions are indicated, then, when the patient's physical or mental condition may be improved by their application. Interventions may be nonindicated for a variety of reasons. First, the intervention may have no scientifically demonstrated effect on the disease to be treated and yet be erroneously selected by the clinician or desired by the patient. An example of such an intervention would be high-dose chemotherapy followed by bone marrow transplantation for widely metastatic breast cancer or the use of estrogens for a postmenopausal woman in the mistaken belief that it will decrease the risk of coronary artery disease. These treatments are nonindicated. Second, an intervention known to be efficacious in general may not have the usual effect in some patients because of individual differences in constitution or in the disease. An example of this type of intervention would be a patient who takes a cholesterol-lowering statin drug and subsequently experiences an acute myopathy, a rare but known serious complication. Statins are not indicated for this patient. Third, an intervention appropriate at one time in the patient's course may cease to be appropriate at a later time. An example of this would be ventilatory support, indicated when a patient is admitted to the hospital after cardiac arrest but no longer indicated when the patient is determined to have profound anoxic brain damage and suffers multisystem organ failure.

This last situation occurs when a patient is so seriously ill or injured that sound clinical judgment would suggest that the goals of restoration of health and function are unattainable and, thus, certain medical interventions that usually perform these functions are not indicated or should be limited. These cases present themselves in several ways: the dying patient, the terminal patient, and the patient with progressive, lethal disease. We illustrate these three conditions by following the case of Mr. Care.

CASE. Mr. Care, a 44-year-old married man with two adult children, was diagnosed as having MS 15 years ago. During the past 12 years, the patient has experienced progressive deterioration and has not responded to the drugs currently approved to delay progression of MS. He is now confined to a wheelchair and for the last 2 years has required an indwelling Foley catheter because of an atonic bladder. He is now blind in one eye, with markedly decreased vision in the other. He has been hospitalized several times because of pyelonephritis and urosepsis. In the course of the last year, he has become profoundly depressed, is uncommunicative even with close family, and refuses to leave his bed. During the entire course of his illness, he has refused to discuss the issue of terminal care, saying he found such discussion depressing and discouraging.

Decisions about what treatment is indicated for Mr. Care are influenced by whether he is viewed as a "dying" patient, a terminally ill patient, or as an incurable patient. These three terms are explained below (and also in Topic Three, Section 3.3, where considerations of quality of life are added to medical indications).

1.1.2 The Dying Patient

Many interventions become nonindicated when the patient is about to die. In this section, we use the word *dying* to describe a situation when clinical conditions indicate definitively that the patient's organ systems are disintegrating rapidly and irreversibly. Death can be expected within hours. This condition is sometimes described as "actively dying" or "imminently dying." In this situation, indications for medical intervention change significantly. We return to the case of Mr. Care.

CASE. Mr. Care, in the advanced stages of MS, suffers from deep decubitus ulcers and osteomyelitis, neither of which has responded to treatment efforts, including skin grafts. During the past month, the patient has been admitted three times to the intensive care unit (ICU) with aspiration pneumonia and has required mechanical ventilation. He is admitted again, requiring ventilation and, after 4 days, becomes septic. On the next day, he is noted to have increasingly stiff lungs and poor oxygenation. In several hours, his blood pressure is 60/40 mm Hg and decreasing. He is unresponsive to pressors and volume expanders. His arterial oxygen saturation is 45%. He is anuric, his creatinine is 5.5 mg/dL and rising, and his arterial pH is 6.92. A house officer asks whether ventilation and pressors are futile and should be discontinued.

COMMENT. Mr. Care has multisystem organ failure and is dying. Medical intervention at this point is sometimes called futile, that is, offering no therapeutic benefit to the patient. Judgments about futility are often very controversial and its meaning will be fully discussed below in Section 1.2.2. At this point in Mr. Care's case, the house officer uses the word *futile* in a quite obvious, noncontroversial way: as a shorthand description of *a condition in which physiological systems have deteriorated so drastically that no known medical intervention can reverse the decline.* The judgment of futility in this case approaches certainty. Some commentators use the phrase *physiological futility* for this situation, and some believe that it is the only situation in which the word *futility* should be applied.

RECOMMENDATION. Mr. Care is dying. His death will take place within hours. Ventilation and vasopressors are no longer indicated, because they are now having no positive physiological effect. *Physiologic futility is an ethical justification for the physician to recommend withdrawing all interventions, with the exception of those that may provide comfort.* If the patient's family requests continued interventions, see the discussion in Section 1.2.2.

1.1.3 The Terminally Ill Patient

Judgments about whether certain interventions are indicated must be reevaluated when a patient is in a terminal condition. There is no standard clinical definition of *terminal*. The word is often loosely used to refer to the prognosis of any patient with a lethal disease. In the Medicare and Medicaid eligibility rules for reimbursement of hospice care, *terminal* is defined as a prediction having 6 months or less to live. This is an administrative rather than a clinical definition. In clinical medicine, *terminal* should be applied *only* to those patients whom experienced clinicians expect will die from a lethal, progressive disease, despite appropriate treatment, in a relatively short period, measured in days, weeks, or several months at most. Diagnosis of a terminal condition should be based on medical evidence and clinical judgment that the condition is progressive, irreversible, and lethal. The benefits of accurate prognostication include informing patients and families about the situation, allowing them to plan their remaining time and arrange appropriate forms of care. However, such prognostication must be made with great caution. More than a few studies have shown that even experienced clinicians often fail to make accurate prognoses. Some physicians are overly pessimistic, but one major study shows that even more clinicians are inappropriately optimistic and fail to inform patients of their imminent death.

Christakis N. *Death Foretold: Prophecy and Prognosis in Medical Care.* Chicago, IL: University of Chicago Press; 1999.

CASE. Prior to the hospitalization described above, Mr. Care is living at home. He requires assistance in all activities of daily life and is confined to bed. He has become confused and disoriented. He begins to experience breathing difficulties and is brought to the emergency department. He is now unresponsive and has a high fever and labored, shallow respirations. A chest radiograph reveals diffuse haziness suggestive of adult respiratory distress syndrome; arterial blood gases show a Po_2 of 35, Pco_2 of 85, and pH of 7.02. Cardiac studies demonstrate an acute anteroseptal myocardial infarction. Neurologic and pulmonary consultants agree that he has primary neuromuscular respiratory insufficiency. Mr Care's family calls his personal physician, who immediately consults with the emergency physicians. Should Mr. Care be intubated and admitted to the ICU? Should his acute myocardial infarction be treated with emergency angioplasty and stenting, or are these procedures not indicated in this patient's condition?

COMMENT. This acute episode is a life-threatening event superimposed upon a chronic, lethal, and deteriorating condition. Various interventions might delay Mr. Care's demise. A respirator may improve gas exchange and support perfusion of organ systems; fibrinolytic therapy or angioplasty plus stenting might limit the evolving infarct. These interventions aim at two of the goals of medicine: support of compromised function and prolongation of life. Given the presence of progressive and irreversible disease in its final stages and radical damage to multiple organ systems, none of the other important goals can be achieved. The patient will certainly never be restored to health, and compromised functions will not be restored but sustained temporarily by mechanical means. The following reflections are relevant:

(a) Mr. Care, now unresponsive, has declined to express preferences about the course of his care, and nothing is known from other sources about his preferences. Therefore, personal preferences, usually so important in these decisions, are not available to clinicians or to surrogates. Objective data about survival and sound clinical discretion about the probabilities of improvement are the most important factors in formulating a recommendation to forgo further treatment.

(b) Objective information that provides prognostic criteria may be useful in determining whether a particular type of intervention will be efficacious. Such objective information may include the patient's diagnosis, physiologic condition, functional status, nutritional status, and comorbidities, together with the patient's estimated likelihood of recovery. One approach to developing these data for patients admitted to the ICU is the Acute Physiology and Chronic Health Evaluation (APACHE). This system combines an acute physiologic score, the Glasgow Coma Score, age, and a chronic disease score to estimate a patient's risk of dying during an ICU admission. Another new and simpler system, Modified Organ Dysfunction Score (MODS), records how many organ systems are dysfunctional and for how many days. Analyses such as these, done for this patient with pneumonia, ARDS, and acute MI, would show that the probability of his surviving this ICU admission is extremely low. Even though probability is not equivalent to certainty, in this instance, as everywhere else in medicine, it is a sound basis for clinical judgment.

(c) In these clinical circumstances, the principle of beneficence, in its sense of helping to remedy the conditions that are leading to death, is no longer applicable. In the absence of patient preferences, quality of life and appropriate use of resources become appropriate ethical considerations; see Topics Three, "Quality of Life," and Four, "Contextual Features."

(d) A medical judgment that none of the goals of medicine can be achieved apart from sustaining organ function provides the first ethical ground to conclude that further life-sustaining treatment can be omitted. The physician should formulate a recommendation to this effect. In addition to this ethical grounding, consent of the patient or the patient's designated surrogate must be sought, as explained in Topic Two.

1.1.4 The Incurable Patients with Progressive, Lethal Disease

Certain diseases follow a course of gradual and sometimes occult destruction of the body's physiologic processes. Patients who suffer such diseases may experience their effects continually or intermittently, and with varying severity. Eventually, the disease itself or some associated disorder will cause death. Mr. Care illustrates the features of this condition. Multiple sclerosis cannot be cured. Progressive neurologic complications that include spasticity, loss of mobility, neurogenic bladder, respiratory insufficiency, and occasionally dementia are also irreversible. Still, some interventions, such as treatment of infection, can relieve symptoms, maintain some level of function, and prolong life.

CASE. For the first decade after his diagnosis with MS, Mr. Care maintained high spirits. Although he did not like to discuss his disease or its prognosis, he seemed to understand the progressive and lethal nature of his condition. However, in the last few years, he has begun to speak frequently of "getting this over" and has become deeply depressed. He has accepted several trials of antidepressant medications, but these did not improve his mental condition. As serious urinary tract and respiratory infections became more frequent, he grudgingly submitted to treatment.

COMMENT. Patients in this condition are not terminal, even though the disease from which they suffer is incurable. However, they may from time to time experience acute, critical episodes, which, if not treated, will lead to their death. When successfully treated, patients will be restored to their "baseline condition." In a sense, they are, at each episode, "potentially terminal." It may occur to such patients and to their physicians that these critical episodes offer an opportunity to end their progressive decline. Recall the old medical maxim, "Pneumonia is the old person's friend." In such a situation, the issues require a careful review of medical indications, because the patient's prognosis, with or without treatment, must be clearly understood. However, the more important questions concern patient preferences and quality of life. Therefore, the ethical dimensions of such cases will be discussed under Topics Two and Three.

Singer PA, MacDonald N, Tulsky JA. Quality end of life care. In: Singer PA, Viens AM, eds. *The Cambridge Textbook of Bioethics.* New York, NY: Cambridge University Press; 2008:53–57.

1.2 CLINICAL JUDGMENT AND CLINICAL UNCERTAINTY

1.2.1 Question Four—What Are the Probabilities of Success of Various Treatment Options?

In the above cases, judgments about diagnosis and treatment reflect a certain level of certainty or uncertainty. Given the nature of medical science and the particularities of each patient, clinical judgment is never absolutely certain. Clinical medicine was described by Dr. William Osler as "a science of uncertainty and an art of probability." The central task of clinicians is to reduce uncertainty to the extent possible by using clinical data, medical science, and reasoning to reach a diagnosis and propose a plan of care. The process by which a clinician attempts to make consistently good decisions in the face of uncertainty is called *clinical judgment.*

The inevitable uncertainty of clinical judgment can be reduced by the methods of evidence-based medicine, using data from controlled clinical trials, and by the development of practice guidelines, which assist the physician's reasoning through a clinical problem. Although evidence-based medicine and practice guidelines aim to reduce the "uncertainty" and the "probability" of which Osler spoke, some degree of uncertainty always remains, because these methods reach general statistical conclusions that may not fit the real patient who is before the physician.

In addition to uncertainty about data and their interpretation, there will be uncertainty about what action to take in any particular case. This is reflected in such questions as "Now that we have medical evidence about what is possible, what should we do?" "Given all the possibilities, what goals are appropriate for this patient?" These questions cannot be solely answered by clinical data. The ethical principles of beneficence and nonmaleficence reduce the scope of this sort of uncertainty by directing intention and effort away from the wide range of possible diagnoses and treatments and toward the more narrow range most likely to help this patient in these circumstances. However, the ethical principles do not dictate particular clinical decisions. These decisions must be confronted in candid, realistic discussions among clinicians, the patient, and the family. This is the shared decision making that constitutes an appropriate professional relationship; see Topic Two, "Patient Preferences."

Feinstein AR. *Clinical Judgment*. New York, NY: Krieger; 1974.
Goodman KW. *Ethics and Evidence-Based Medicine. Fallibility and Responsibility in Clinical Science*. Cambridge, MA: Cambridge University Press; 2003.

1.2.2 Medical Futility

An important ethical problem is closely associated with the probabilistic nature of medical judgment. The question is whether a high probability that a particular treatment will be unsuccessful justifies withholding or withdrawing that treatment. This is often called the *futility problem*, or "medically ineffective or nonbeneficial treatment." A long, hotly contested debate over "futility" has been inconclusive. One definition at the center of the debate states: "futility designates an effort to provide a benefit to a patient, which reason and experience suggest is highly likely to fail and whose rare exceptions cannot be systematically produced." In Section 1.1.2, we have seen the term "physiologic futility," that is, an utter impossibility that the desired physiologic response can be affected by any intervention. However, *futility* more properly is a judgment about probabilities, and its accuracy depends on empirical data drawn from clinical studies and from clinical experience. Because clinical studies that demonstrate this sort of futility are rare, and because clinical experience is so varied, clinicians make widely different estimates of futility: physicians' judgments that various procedures should be called futile range from 0% to 50% chance of success, clustering about 10%. Some ethicists and clinicians deny the utility of the concept of futility because of its confused meaning and frequently inappropriate application. Others, including ourselves, consider it a useful term when applied thoughtfully to treatment decisions about interventions with low likelihood of success.

Beauchamp TL, Childress JF. Conditions for overriding the prima facie obligation to treat. In: Beauchamp L, Childress JF, eds. *Principles of Biomedical Ethics*. 6th ed. New York, NY: Oxford University Press; 2009:167–169.

Lo B. Futile interventions. In: Lo B, ed. *Resolving Ethical Dilemmas. A Guide for Physicians*. 4th ed. Philadelphia, PA: Lippincott Williams & Wilkins; 2009:61–66.

Schneiderman LJ, Jecker NS, Jonsen AR. Medical futility: its meaning, and ethical implications. *Ann Intern Med*. 1990;112:949–954.

Three main questions about futility are debated: (1) What level of statistical or experiential evidence is required to support a judgment of futility? (2) Who decides whether an intervention is futile, physicians or patients? (3) What process should be used to resolve disagreements between patients (or their surrogates) and the medical team about whether a particular treatment is futile?

(1) *Statistical probability*. Clinical futility requires a probabilistic judgment that an intervention is highly unlikely to produce the desired result. This judgment comes from general clinical experience and from clinical studies that demonstrate low rates of success for particular interventions, such as CPR for certain types of patients, or continued ventilatory support for patients with adult respiratory disease syndrome. Even the data that are available may prove deceptive in a particular case because studies apply to groups rather than individuals. Further, a lack of agreement exists about how low a level of probability would justify calling a treatment futile. One group has suggested that if soundly designed clinical studies reveal less than a 1% chance of success, intervention should be considered futile.

EXAMPLE I. A study of 865 patients who required mechanical ventilation after bone marrow transplantation showed no survivors among the 383 patients who had lung injury or hepatic or renal failure and who required more than 4 hours of ventilator support. This study suggests that it would be probabilistically futile to intubate patients with these conditions or to continue ventilation after 4 hours.

Rubenfeld GD, Crawford SW. Withdrawing life support for medically ventilated recipients of bone marrow transplantation: a case for evidence-based qualitative guidelines. *Ann Intern Med*. 1996;125:625–633.

EXAMPLE II. A large clinical study examined hospital discharge records of more than 5000 patients from eight U.S. cities, who suffered cardiac arrest out of hospital, were resuscitated by emergency teams, and were transported to hospital for further care. The investigators applied rules they had developed earlier for stopping CPR in the field and then tried to predict which of the resuscitated patients would survive to be discharged from the hospital. Their study was designed to validate the rules for predicting CPR futility. None of the 1192 patients who did not meet Advanced Life Support criteria for termination of CPR survived to discharge; of 776 patients who met Basic Life Support criteria, 4 (0.5%) survived to discharge.

Sasson C, Hegg AJ, Macy M, et al. Prehospital termination of resuscitation in cases of refractory out-of-hospital cardiac arrest. *JAMA*. 2008;12:1432–1438.

COMMENT. The first study was done in 1996. It clearly illustrates probabilistic futility: not a single patient from a large cohort left the ICU alive. A decade later, these data have not been contradicted. The second study was a retrospective cohort study developed to predict when it would be futile to continue resuscitation in cases of refractory out-of-hospital cardiac arrest. Applying these rules to the data accurately predicted 99.9% of the patients who did not survive to hospital discharge. Therefore, these rules predicted probabilistic futility in out-of-hospital cardiac arrests with great accuracy.

(2) *Who decides?* It is relatively rare that carefully designed clinical studies such as the previous reports provide hard data for determination of futility. Inevitable debates will ensue about the level of probability that should represent futility. Who has the authority to establish the goals of the intervention and to decide the level of probability for attaining such goals? Some ethicists argue that physicians have the right to refuse care that they believe is highly unlikely to produce beneficial results; other ethicists maintain that futility must be defined in light of the subjective views, values, and goals of patients and their surrogates.

CASE I. A 75-year-old woman is brought to the ER by paramedics after suffering massive head trauma, with extrusion of brain tissue, as a result of a vehicular accident. She had been intubated by the paramedics. After careful evaluation, the ER physicians judged that her injuries were so severe that no intervention could retard her imminent death. When her grieving family gather in the ER, they demand that the woman be admitted to the ICU and be prepared for operation by a neurosurgeon. The physicians state that further treatment is futile.

CASE II. Helga Wanglie was an elderly Minnesota woman who suffered irreversible brain damage from strokes and slipped into a chronic vegetative state. She required mechanical ventilation. Physicians and family agreed that she had no hope of regaining the ability to interact with others. However, Mrs. Wanglie's husband refused to authorize discontinuing the ventilator, saying that his goal (and, he asserted, hers) was that her life should not be shortened, regardless of her prospects for neurologic recovery. Physicians requested court intervention to authorize withdrawal of ventilatory support.

CASE III. A 72-year-old man with late-stage emphysema is admitted to the ICU with fever, respiratory failure, and hypoxemia. While he is being intubated, he has a cardiac arrest. He is resuscitated in the unit, but remains unconscious after resuscitation. He is found to have had a large anterior wall myocardial infarction, requiring pressors to maintain blood pressure. The laboratory calls to say that blood culture data drawn in the ER are growing gram-negative bacteria. Because of his multisystem organ failure and sepsis, the physicians decide to write a DNR order, believing that a second attempt at CPR would be futile.

COMMENT. In Case I, the physicians are speaking of futility in the sense used in Section 1.1.2, that is, physiological futility. The issue here is not the likelihood but the impossibility of continued life regardless of any intervention. They are ethically justified in refusing to pursue treatment. In Case II, continued ventilatory support and other interventions can extend Mrs. Wanglie's life. These interventions, employed for this purpose, cannot be judged physiologically futile. However, physicians judge that there is a vanishingly low probability of restoring Mrs. Wanglie's health and a low probability also that her life will be extended very long, even with support. They also judge that Mrs. Wanglie's life, if extended, will be of very low quality. Physicians may recommend termination of the intervention on the grounds of medical futility, but they lack the ethical authority to define the benefit of continued life even without consciousness. This is a matter for the patient and her surrogate to decide (as the Minnesota court determined). Some contextual features, such as scarcity of resources, might be relevant to this case (see Topic Four, "Contextual Features," Section 4.5).

In Case III, the patient's multiorgan system failure, dependence on pressors, and sepsis make it highly unlikely that a second resuscitation will succeed. A DNR order should be recommended to appropriate surrogates.

(3) *Dispute Resolution.* What process should be used to resolve disputes about futility? Institutions should design a policy for conflict resolution. These policies should prohibit unilateral decision making by physicians, except in cases of physiological futility. For judgments of futility based on low probability of successful treatment, policy should stress the need for valid empirical evidence, provide for consultation with outside

experts and with ethics committees, and, above all, create an atmosphere of open negotiation or mediation rather than confrontation. The policy should allow physicians to withdraw from cases in which they judge continued treatment futile and should provide for transfer of patients to other institutions willing to accept them. Futility arguments should be moved into court only after all other reasonable attempts to resolve the disagreement fail. Elements of a model hospital policy on nonbeneficial care can be found in the *AMA Code of Medical Ethics* 2008, 2.037 (www.ama-assn.org).

COMMENT. Despite continued debates about the concept of futility, we believe it is useful in medical ethics, because it highlights the necessity to make decisions about treatments that are of questionable benefit. It introduces a note of realism into excessive medical optimism by inviting physicians and families to focus on what realistically can be done for the patient under the circumstances and which goals, if any, can be realized. It provides the opportunity to open an honest discussion with patients and their families about appropriate care. It calls for a careful investigation of the literature about the efficacy of proposed treatments in particular situations.

Physicians should never invoke futility, except in the sense of physiologic futility, to justify unilateral decision making or to avoid a difficult conversation with patient or family. A physician's judgment that further treatment would be futile does not justify a conclusion that treatment should cease; instead, it signals that discussions of the situation with patient and family are mandatory. Futility should never be invoked when the real problem is a frustration with a difficult case or a reflection of the physician's negative evaluation of the patient's future quality of life; see Topic Three, "Quality of Life." Also, a futility claim by itself does not justify rules or guidelines devised by third-party payers to avoid paying for care; see Topic Four, "Contextual Features." Further, even when the facts of the case support a judgment of futility, we suggest that it may be advisable to avoid the actual word "futility" in discussions with patients or their families. Many persons may interpret this word as an announcement that the physician is "giving up" on the patient or that the patient is not worth further attention. At this point, rather than explicitly using futility language, clinicians should raise the question of redirecting the efforts of clinical care to palliation and comfort, because the burdens of more aggressive care far exceed the chances for benefit. Ethicists sometimes refer to this reasoning as *proportionality* (see Section 3.3.5).

Finally, we acknowledge that a physician has the moral right to withdraw from a case in which he or she has reached an honest judgment of futility, even though continued care is demanded by others. Such a judgment would be based on the belief that nothing is being done to benefit the patient, while continued interventions actually are harming the patient. Should a physician reach this conclusion, proper steps to inform the family should be taken. Hospital policy should support physician's judgments in this regard.

1.3 CARDIOPULMONARY RESUSCITATION (CPR) AND ORDERS NOT TO RESUSCITATE (DNR)

The practice of CPR provides another example in which estimations of the probability of success are often a crucial element of the ethical decision to proceed with the intervention. *Cardiopulmonary resuscitation consists of a set of techniques designed to restore circulation and respiration in the event of acute cardiac or cardiopulmonary arrest.* The most common causes of cardiac arrest are (1) cardiac arrhythmia, (2) acute respiratory insufficiency, and (3) hypotension. The omission of CPR after cardiopulmonary arrest will result in the death of the patient.

Basic CPR, consisting of mouth-to-mouth ventilation and chest compression, is taught to lay persons for use in emergency situations. Automatic defibrillation devices are now available for lay use as well. In hospitals, advanced CPR is usually done by a trained team who respond to an urgent call. Advanced CPR techniques include closed-chest compression, intubation with assisted ventilation, electroconversion of arrhythmias, and use of cardiotonic and vasopressive drugs.

CPR is an indicated procedure to reverse the effects of cardiopulmonary arrest. However, it is not indicated when a clinical judgment is made that the procedure is unlikely to do so. Therefore, clinicians must recognize situations in which low probability of success dictates a decision to refrain from CPR.

The Joint Commission requires that hospitals have an explicit policy regarding CPR. Since the 1960s, those policies have required that CPR be a standing order, that is, CPR is to be performed on any patient who suffers a cardiac or respiratory arrest without needing any written order for the procedure. The policies require that an order be written to authorize *omission* of CPR for a particular patient. Thus, in contrast to every other hospital procedure, clinicians may withhold CPR only when a specific order states that it should be omitted. This order is designated Do-Not-Resuscitate (DNR) and is frequently called a "No Code Order."

Questions have been raised about the standard policy requiring resuscitation except when a specific order authorizes its omission. Some commentators believe that decisions to resuscitate should be an affirmative order based on medical indications and patient preferences. We agree with this position.

Under the present policies, however, the decision to write a DNR order should be based on two crucial considerations. The first is the judgment that CPR is not medically indicated in the case, that is, not likely to restore physiological function; it will be futile, in the sense explained in Section 1.2.2. The second consideration is the permission of the patient or of the designated surrogate. The medical futility of the intervention will be treated here; patient preferences, surrogate decisions, and quality of life will be discussed in Topics Two and Three.

Lo B. Do not attempt resuscitation orders. In: Lo B, ed. *Resolving Ethical Dilemmas. A Guide for Physicians*. 3rd ed. Philadelphia, PA: Lippincott Williams & Wilkins; 2005:111–116.

Sanders AB. Emergency and trauma medical ethics. In: Singer PA, Viens AM, eds. *The Cambridge Textbook of Bioethics*. Cambridge: Cambridge University Press; 2008:469–474.

1.3.1 Medical Indications and Contraindications for CPR

All hospitalized patients who suffer unexpected cardiopulmonary arrest should be resuscitated unless the following occurs:

(a) There is conclusive evidence that the patient is dead, such as rigor mortis, exsanguination, or decapitation (physiological futility).
(b) No physiological benefit can be expected, because the patient has deteriorated despite maximal therapy for such conditions as progressive sepsis or multisystem organ failure (probabilistic futility).
(c) The patient has a valid DNR order.

International Resuscitation Guidelines 2000. Part 2: Ethical Aspects of CPR and ECC. Criteria for Not Starting CPR. *Resuscitation*. 2000;46(1–3):17–27.

COMMENT

(a) Cardiopulmonary resuscitation is not indicated when cardiopulmonary arrest occurs as the anticipated end of a terminal illness, and when all treatment options have failed. Because cardiopulmonary arrest is the most frequent cause of death for such patients, a DNR order should be written.

(b) DNR orders are usually first considered when the patient is in a terminal condition and death appears to be imminent. A multicenter study of DNR orders in ICUs showed that fewer than 2% of patients who had DNR orders survived to be discharged from the hospital. These patients are often imminently dying, and thus highly unlikely to benefit from CPR. In such cases, the DNR order allows the patient to die without burdensome resuscitative efforts. This achieves the medical goal of a peaceful death.

(c) In the United States, the rate of DNR orders varies from 3% to 30% among hospitalized patients and between 5% and 20% among patients admitted to ICUs. Sixty-six percent to 75% of hospital deaths and 40% of deaths in ICUs are preceded by a DNR order. Even after adjusting for severity of illness, disparities exist in the use of DNR orders relative to age, race, gender, and geography. Older patients, white patients, and women are more likely to have DNR orders. Some geographic areas have a DNR rate 8 to 10 times higher than that of others.

Wenger NS, Pearson ML, Desmond KA, et al. Epidemiology of do-not-resuscitate orders: disparity by age, diagnosis, gender, race, and functional impairment. *Arch Intern Med.* 1995;155(19):2056–2062.

(d) Studies show that the success of CPR varies with different types of patients. Survival after CPR was more likely in the following situations: (1) for patients with respiratory rather than cardiac arrest; (2) for witnessed cardiac arrests, initial ventricular tachycardia, or fibrillation; (3) for patients with no or few comorbid conditions; (4) for cardiac arrest caused by readily identifiable iatrogenic causes; and (5) for patients who experience a short duration of arrest. Survival is much less likely in patients with preexisting hypotension, renal failure, sepsis, pneumonia, acute stroke, metastatic cancer, or a homebound lifestyle. One large study of patients older than 65 years who were resuscitated in hospital showed a survival to discharge of 18.3%, with survival rates lower for men, older patients, patients with comorbidities. Survival for black patients was 23.6% lower than for whites.

Ehlenbah WJ, Barnato AE, Curtis JR. Epidemiologic study of in-hospital cardiopulmonary resuscitation in the elderly. *N Engl J Med.* 2009;361:22–31.

(e) Among patients who experience in-hospital cardiac arrest and who are resuscitated, 10% to 17% survive to hospital discharge. For those patients who survive to discharge, several studies have shown good prognosis, with long-term survival rates of 33% to 54%. Patients who experience cardiac arrest outside the hospital have a 3% to 14% chance of survival to discharge. Among patients who survive arrest in either setting, 11% to 14% have some neurologic impairment at discharge and 26% have some restriction on activities of daily living.

(f) Studies also indicate that even for terminally ill patients, DNR orders are underused, as demonstrated by the disparity between the number of patients who had indicated a preference for such orders in relation to those for whom orders were actually written. Presumably, this happens because of a lack of communication and discussion among physicians, patients, and their families. In our view, physicians have an ethical responsibility to initiate DNR discussions in the following situations: (1) with patients who are terminally ill or patients who have an incurable disease with an estimated 50% survival of less than 3 years; (2) with all patients who suffer acute, life-threatening conditions; and (3) with all patients who request such a discussion. When patients are incapable of discussing DNR orders, physicians should have such discussions with the patients' surrogate.

(g) Patients and families often overestimate the success of CPR. This misapprehension may be fostered by media versions of CPR. A study of cardiac resuscitation on television hospital dramas showed that 67% of televised "patients" survived, in contrast to the much lower numbers in "real" clinical situations. Also, many patients have little idea of the nature of resuscitation procedures and, when informed of them, often choose not to have resuscitation. It is essential that patients, their families, and physicians have accurate information on the benefits and risks of CPR so that they can make informed decisions about using CPR or choosing DNR status.

Diem SJ, Lantos JD, Tulsky JA. Cardiopulmonary resuscitation on television. Miracles and misinformation. *N Engl J Med.* 1996;334(24):1578–1582.

(h) DNR orders apply only to decisions about refraining from cardiopulmonary resuscitation and should not influence decisions about interventions other than CPR. DNR orders are often written when doctors, patients, and surrogates intend to withhold or withdraw other life-prolonging treatments. When this is the case, distinct orders should be written specifying which treatments other than CPR should be withheld and under what circumstances.

CASE. Mr. Care, the patient with MS, has been admitted to the hospital in coma for treatment of pneumonia and respiratory failure. In the past, he has emphasized to his family and physicians that he did not wish to be placed on permanent mechanical ventilation. Neurologic consultation concludes that his respiratory insufficiency is secondary to the advancing muscular and neurologic deterioration of MS and that respiratory failure was accelerated by his acute pneumonia. Should a DNR order be written?

RECOMMENDATIONS. In the case of Mr. Care, recommendations should be made to the family that even if CPR succeeds, the patient would survive only a short time without permanent ventilatory support. Based on the patient's prior wishes not to be permanently intubated, a DNR order should be recommended. If the family concurs, a DNR order should be entered. If the family disagrees, an ethics review is mandatory because the family's decision to resuscitate is in conflict with the patient's own previously expressed wishes not to be on mechanical ventilation.

COMMENT. Decisions to recommend DNR orders are obviously dependent on the clinical situation of each patient. For the immanently dying patient, the very low probability of success supports DNR. For other terminally ill patients, the combination of factors, such as comorbidities and age, must be taken into account in calculating the probability of success (see Sections 1.1.2, 1.1.3, and 3.3). In all cases, it is essential to recognize that CPR is not an innocuous intervention: it can cause serious bruising, broken bones, etc. Also, even if initially successful, another arrest may follow, instigating another resuscitation. Finally, intubation may initiate a life-support situation that itself may generate an ethical problem of futility. Therefore, the most careful evaluation of a patient's likelihood of being successfully resuscitated and of being discharged from the hospital is an essential component of an ethical decision to refrain from resuscitation.

1.3.2 Patient Choice of DNR

In addition to terminally ill and dying patients, competent, nonterminally ill patients may initiate discussion of DNR orders with their physicians. For these patients, a DNR order is an important component of advance care planning, allowing them to express preferences about treatment at the end of life, which we discuss more fully in Topic Two. Many of these patients are in the earlier phases of serious diseases, such as metastatic cancer, AIDS, or ALS. They are prepared to forgo resuscitation attempts because they are concerned that even if they are "successfully" resuscitated, they may experience anoxic brain damage or some other functional impairment or go on to live through a painful terminal phase of their illness. Physicians should carefully discuss these requests with the patient and honor them. While very few ICU patients with DNR orders survive to hospital discharge, outcomes for nonterminal, seriously ill patients are much better. Several published studies have shown survival to discharge to be as high as 50% to 70%.

1.3.3 DNR Orders Without or Contrary to Consent

Ordinarily, the consent of the patient or the patient's surrogate is required to write DNR orders. Three situations raise questions about this general rule. (a) A patient may be unable to give consent and no surrogate can be identified. (b) Medical indications may not support the utility of CPR, but surrogates insist that it be done. (c) In an emergency crisis, when survival is highly unlikely. *Medical ethicists are divided on the question whether it is ever ethically acceptable for a physician to make a unilateral decision, that is, a decision not to resuscitate without the consent of the patient or the patient's surrogate, perhaps even in the face of objections from the patient or surrogate.* Those in favor of unilateral decisions argue that no medical procedure that is not indicated, that is, unlikely to effect a positive change in the patient's condition, should be performed. Further, they argue that CPR performed in these situations can cause great distress to the patient, adding to the burdens of immanent death. Finally, they note that even a successful resuscitation in the crisis would likely lead to another crisis and another resuscitation attempt, ad infinitum. In such a situation, a physician, they say, should have the right to give a DNR order even without patient or surrogate consent. Those who oppose unilateral decisions maintain that the patient should always have the right to refuse or choose CPR, because a decision about the goals of treatment and the acceptable probability of attaining those goals is a value judgment only the patient can make. Depending on the patient's goals, even the remote chance of successful resuscitation may be of value to the patient. These critics also assert that the concept of futility is too vague to be consistently applied. Critics of unilateral DNR also warn that such decisions are open to bias against patients at risk of discrimination (see Section 3.1.1).

COMMENT. If the physician has concluded that CPR has no prospect of resuscitating the patient, the physician may recommend that CPR be withheld. If the patient is unable to consent to this recommendation, and no surrogate is available, a DNR order may be written on the basis of futility. If patient or surrogates refuse the recommendation, the physician should seek a second medical opinion about the futility or utility of resuscitation. The "two doctor rule" is frequently misunderstood. The opinion of a second physician is not equivalent to permission or consent to DNR; it is simply a confirmation of the first clinical opinion that resuscitation would be unlikely to benefit the patient. Serious attempts to reconcile differences of opinion should be undertaken. An ethics consultation should be sought. If no agreement can be reached, the hospital policy on nonbeneficial care should be invoked (see Section 1.2.2). We do not believe that a physician has the right to make a unilateral decision to write a DNR order.

A physician may, however, refrain from resuscitation when an arrest occurs, or is likely to occur, in a critical situation in which it is apparent that the patient's survival, under any circumstances, is highly unlikely. Therefore, patients arriving in the ER with extreme traumatic injuries, or after being found down for an extended period of time, need not be resuscitated.

1.3.4 Documentation of DNR Orders

Code status should be clear to all who have responsibility for the patient, particularly nurses and house officers. Attending physicians should clearly write and sign the DNR order in the patient's chart. The progress notes should include the medical facts and opinion underlying the order and a summary of the discussion with the patient, consultants, staff, and family. Some clear sign of the DNR status should be affixed to the chart, such as a green dot. The status of the order should be changed if the condition of the patient warrants it. Everyone involved with the care of the patient should be informed of the DNR order and its rationale. Because studies have shown that DNR means different things to different practitioners, the physician writing the order must be careful to document the specific terms of the order. The writing of a DNR order should have no direct bearing on any treatment other than CPR. If a DNR order has not been written, the patient is presumed to be "full code." Code status should be reevaluated at each hospital admission.

1.3.5 DNR Portability

Patients for whom DNR orders have been written in the hospital may be discharged with the expectation that they will die soon. Often, patients want to die in their own homes rather than in the hospital. Family members sometimes summon emergency services if these patients suffer a crisis at home. Traditionally, emergency medical service providers, because of the time constraints inherent in emergency services, were not responsible for determining whether a patient had an advance directive. They attempted to resuscitate all patients regardless of the patients' preferences. In recent years, a method of protecting an individual's preference not to be resuscitated has been devised. This is called a "portable" DNR. These are orders issued by the patient's discharging physician, stated in a standard form, and indicated on bracelets, necklaces, or wallet cards. When the patient has this order, emergency technicians are authorized to refrain from CPR, although all other necessary treatments can still be provided. Almost every state now has laws or regulations mandating that EMS providers comply with out-of-hospital DNRs. Once the emergency care provider has verified that the order appears valid and that the patient is the person who has executed it, the provider cannot commence CPR except in certain circumstances, such as when the patient renounces the document.

1.3.6 POLST Orders (Physicians Orders for Life-Sustaining Treatment)

The POLST paradigm is a physician's order form that contains a summary of a patient's choices about the nature and extent of life-sustaining procedures that they wish to have done or omitted. The form contains four sections—A: Cardiopulmonary Resuscitation; B: Medical Interventions, that is, comfort measures only, limited interventions or full treatment; C: artificially administered nutrition; and D: summary of medical condition. POLST is a physician order and is signed by the physician. But unlike most physician orders, it is also signed by the patient or the surrogate. It should be a part of the patient's hospital record. The primary purpose of POLST is to record all the patient's wishes in a single document and ensure that these wishes follow the patient across different health care settings, for example, from the acute care hospital to a skilled nursing facility. When suitable state law and regulation allows, emergency medical personnel, as well as other providers, may honor the POLST directives. As of 2010, Washington, Oregon, California, West Virginia, North Carolina, Tennessee, and New York have recognized POLST.

1.3.7 "Slow Codes" and "Partial Codes"

The term "slow code" describes a subterfuge in which doctors and nurses respond slowly to a cardiac arrest and perform CPR without energy or enthusiasm to pretend that something is being done. This might be done in two circumstances: (1) when the medical team feels that resuscitation would be futile, but no discussion has taken place with the patient or the family, or (2) when the family has chosen resuscitation, although the team feels it would be useless. Some clinicians justify the "slow code" by suggesting that it assuages the guilt of a family who are distressed that they have not "done everything" for their loved one. A slow code is crass dissimulation and unethical.

The expression "partial code" or "chemical code" refers to the practice of separating the various interventions that constitute resuscitation and using them selectively; for example, chest compression, assisted breathing by resuscitator bag, and cardiotonic drugs may be ordered, but electrocardioversion and intubation may be omitted. Although there may be occasional justification for such a procedure, it must be recognized that what is being done is not cardiopulmonary resuscitation in the proper sense. In our view, CPR is an integral procedure of several constituents and all these constituents should be applied unless a patient has clearly expressed preferences to the contrary.

1.3.8 DNR Orders in the Operating Room

Patients may suffer a cardiac arrest in the course of a surgical intervention. In such cases, anesthesiologists immediately initiate resuscitation. Occasionally, patients for whom a DNR order has been written, such as patients with terminal cancer, may require a palliative surgical procedure, such as emergency relief of a bowel obstruction to relieve pain or the elective insertion of a gastrostomy tube or a central venous catheter. The question is whether the DNR order should be suspended automatically during anesthesia or surgery so that resuscitation would be performed if the patient experienced a perioperative cardiac arrest.

The arguments favoring automatic suspension of DNR are as follows: (1) anesthesia and surgery place patients at risk for cardiac and hemodynamic instability; (2) most arrests in the operating room are reversible, because skilled personnel and equipment are at hand; (3) in consenting to surgery, the patient can be assumed to give implied consent for resuscitation; and (4) surgeons and anesthesiologists should not be prevented from treating potentially reversible situations, especially because they do not wish deaths of terminally ill patients to be considered surgical deaths when standard resuscitative techniques have been prohibited. In one study, the majority of anesthesiologists assumed that DNR was implicitly suspended during surgery, and only half of anesthesiologists discussed this assumption with the patient or the surrogate.

Those opposed to automatic suspension of DNR orders note that such a policy ignores patients' rights and violates the standards of informed consent. Critics of automatic suspension deny that consent of the patient should be "implied." They suggest that a terminally ill patient may welcome a perioperative arrest as relief from a painful death. They recommend a policy of "required reconsideration." The patient who consents to elective surgery faces a different risk–benefit situation, and this merits a reevaluation of the DNR order. A specific discussion about DNR should occur between the attending physicians and surgeons and the patient or surrogates. As the result of this discussion, the DNR order should either be affirmed or suspended in anticipation of surgery. The major professional associations of surgeons, anesthesiologists, and nurses have endorsed this policy, and we recommend it as the most prudent course. A surgeon or anesthesiologist may withdraw from a case if he or she judges that failure to resuscitate intraoperatively is unethical.

Another approach to this problem is to develop DNR orders that list the goals of the patient and that permit the surgeon and anesthesiologist to use their clinical judgment to try to achieve the patient's goals. Therefore, if the patient fears anoxic brain damage and experiences ventricular tachycardia that is promptly corrected by cardioversion, the patient's goal of avoiding brain damage will be met. Alternatively, if the patient experiences 15 or more minutes of cardiac arrest, secondary to an intraoperative MI, the surgeon and the anesthesiologist may stop CPR to respect the patient's wish not to survive with neurologic damage.

Statement of the American College of Surgeons. Advance directive by patients: do not resuscitate in the operating room. *Bull Am Coll Surg.* 1994;79(9):29.
Van Norman G. Anesthesiology ethics. In: Singer PA, Viens AM, eds. *The Cambridge Textbook of Bioethics*. New York, NY: Cambridge University Press; 2008:454–461.

1.4 MEDICAL ERROR

Physicians not only work under uncertainty, but they also make mistakes. An Institute of Medicine report (1999) on medical error estimated that between 44,000 and 98,000 Americans die each year as a result of medical errors—more than the number who die from vehicular accidents or from breast cancer or AIDS. In that report, *error* was defined as the failure of a planned action to be completed as intended, or as the use of a wrong plan to achieve an aim. The report highlighted the personal and financial costs of error and noted that some errors were due to incompetence or errors of judgment by competent physicians. Other errors were caused by system failures that often went unrecognized and uncorrected. Following the IOM report, serious efforts have been launched to reduce medical error by increased reporting and analysis of error, by focusing on hospital safety through use of computerized orders and medical records, by establishing patient safety indicators, and by attempting to alleviate the effects of fatigue for house staff and nurses.

Our definition of medical error is an unintentional lapse in a process usually done efficiently and effectively due to (1) inadequate information and/or (2) mistaken judgment and/or (3) defective maneuvers that may or may not be negligent, and may or may not cause harm. Every instance of presumptive error should be analyzed in terms of these elements. It is most important to determine whether or not the error was due to negligence, that is, a performance that peers in a specialty would judge as a departure from accepted standards of practice. Medical error raises ethical problems related to truth telling, which will be discussed at Section 2.1.11. Systemic error describes clinical systems or record-keeping systems that, due to unclarity or inadequacy, lead clinicians to make mistakes. For example, the abbreviation "u" to designate "units of insulin" can easily be read as "0," such that 10 units is read as 100 units. Systematic error is an issue of organizational ethics: "u" is now generally a disapproved symbol in prescription writing. Organizational ethics is discussed in Topic Four, at Section 4.11.

Institute of Medicine. *To Err Is Human: Building a Safer Health System.* Washington, DC: National Academy Press; 1999.

1.5 DETERMINATION OF DEATH

The obligation to provide medical intervention ceases when the patient is declared dead. Declaring death is one of the legal duties of physicians. Traditionally, the moment of death was considered to be the time when a person ceased, and did not resume, communication, movement, and breathing. The body soon becomes cold and rigid, and putrefaction sets in. Physicians customarily determined death by noting the absence of respiration and pulse and the fixation of pupils. Thus, the common definition of death, accepted in medicine and in the law, was "irreversible cessation of circulation and respiration." This is known as the "cardiorespiratory criterion" of death.

This criterion presupposes loss of the integrating function of the brainstem. When this function ceases, spontaneous breathing stops, followed by a disintegration of all vital organ systems. The unoxygenated brain rapidly loses all cognitive and physiologic regulatory functions; the unoxygenated heart ceases to beat. In the 1960s, it became possible to maintain respiratory functions by the use of a mechanical ventilator, which supports oxygen perfusion even in the absence of brainstem function.

The concept of "brain criteria" for death that would complement or replace "cardiorespiratory criteria" emerged in the 1960s. The advent of organ transplantation stimulated interest in this concept, because its application would make possible the preservation of organs within the body after death. In 1968, this concept was clarified in the *Harvard Report on Brain Death*. This report described certain clinical characteristics of a person with a nonfunctioning brain: unreceptivity and unresponsivity to external stimuli, no movements or breathing, no reflexes, and no discernible electrical activity in the cerebral cortex as shown by electroencephalogram (EEG).

The use of "brain criteria" for determination of clinical death was gradually accepted by legal jurisdictions. However, much confusion existed about their proper application. In particular, confusion existed between "total brain death" and "irreversible coma," now called "chronic or continuous vegetative state" (see Section 3.3.3). This confusion was the source of ethical and legal problems. In 1981, the President's Commission for the Study of Ethical Problems in Medicine proposed a model legal statute, the Uniform Definition of Death (UDDA). Every state and the District of Columbia now accept the brain death criteria either by statute or by judicial decision.

> An individual who has sustained either (1) irreversible cessation of circulatory and respiratory function, or (2) irreversible cessation of all functions of the entire brain, including the brain stem, is dead. A determination of death must be made in accordance with accepted medical standards.

President's Commission on Ethical Problems in Medicine and Biomedical and Behavioral Research. *Defining Death: A Report on the Medical, Legal, and Ethical Issues in Definition of Death.* Washington, DC: Government Printing Office; 1981. http://www.bioethics.gov/reports/past_commissions/defining_death.pdf. Accessed November 9, 2009.

The accepted medical standards for clinical diagnosis of death by brain criteria are as follows: after ruling out confounding conditions such as drug intoxication and severe hypothermia, it should be demonstrated that there are no voluntary or involuntary movements except spinal reflexes and no brainstem reflexes; apnea is demonstrated in the presence of elevated arterial CO_2 when mechanical ventilation is temporarily halted, pupils are dilated, fixed at midposition, and there is no reaction to aural irrigation nor gag reflex. Brain blood-flow studies are confirmatory but rarely necessary. Electroencephalography, which diagnoses only the absence of cortical function, is not sufficient to establish total brain death and may be omitted in the presence of the above clinical signs.

No medical goals are attainable for a person who is dead by either cardiorespiratory criteria or brain criteria. No medical interventions are indicated, and all current interventions should be terminated. The physician has the authority to declare the patient dead. There is no legal or ethical requirement to seek permission from the family to declare a patient dead or to discontinue medical interventions. The family should be sensitively informed that their relative has died. Contextual features of a particular case might suggest a continuation of supportive technology, for example, sensitivity to needs of family and friends of the patient, salvage of a viable fetus from a brain-dead pregnant woman, or retrieval of organs for transplant (see Topic Four, "Contextual Features" at Sections 4.2.2; 4.5.7).

Physicians must distinguish the ethical and legal implications of death by brain criteria from the implications of the vegetative state. Lay persons (and some physicians and nurses) use the term *brain death* when they are referring to a vegetative state. This is wrong. Clinicians should use the term *death by brain criteria* when determining death. The ethical and legal implications of a diagnosis of vegetative state are discussed in Section 3.3.3.

Certain philosophical problems about the definition of death by brain criteria remain open to debate. These disputes need not concern those responsible for clinical decisions in this matter. At the present time, physicians in every legal jurisdiction can rely on the legal, clinical, and ethical determinations mentioned earlier. Religious denominations have generally accepted this definition of death. The notable exception is Orthodox

Judaism, where many authorities insist on use of the cardiorespiratory criteria for theological reasons. The State of New Jersey acknowledges this religious exception, allowing surrogates to require cardiorespiratory evidence of death.

Lo B. Determination of death. In: Lo B, ed. *Resolving Ethical Dilemmas. A Guide for Clinicians.* 4th ed. Philadelphia, PA: Lippincott Williams & Wilkins; 2009:143–146.

President's Council on Bioethics. *Controversies in the Determination of Death.* Washington, DC, 2008. http://www.bioethics.gov.

Shemie S, Lazar N, Dickens B. Brain death. In: Singer PA, Viens AM, eds. *The Cambridge Textbook of Bioethics.* New York, NY: Cambridge University Press; 2008:85–94.

Younger S. The definition of death. In: Steinbock B, ed. *The Oxford Handbook of Bioethics.* New York, NY: Oxford University Press; 2009:chap 12.

1.6 SUMMARY

1.6.1 Question Five—In Sum, How Can This Patient Be Benefited by Medical and Nursing Care, and How Can Harm Be Avoided?

This final question for *Medical Indications* moves beyond the gathering and sorting of factual information about the patient's condition and treatment. It requires the clinician to assess how these facts relate to the principles of beneficence and nonmaleficence, and how that assessment can lead to a recommendation about appropriate action. When the clinical facts reveal that a condition is probably treatable, and when benefit–risk reasoning inclines toward intervention, the principles of beneficence and nonmaleficence urge a prudent medical intervention. When, as our discussion of futility shows, the facts favor the opinion that the condition is not amenable to treatment, or when the harm that might occur as a consequence of treatment is significant, the obligation to intervene is diminished, or extinguished. The principle of nonmaleficence then becomes stronger, directing the alleviation of burdens on the patient. Certain benefits of nursing care and palliative treatments remain possible. Finally, as our discussion of death shows, neither benefit nor harm is possible and no intervention whatsoever is indicated.

It must be emphasized that this chapter has dealt with benefit in its objective medical sense, namely, the physical or psychological contributions that will restore a state of health. The clinician's judgments about these objective benefits must now be fashioned into a recommendation offered to the patient for his or her personal consideration and acceptance (or refusal). This is the matter for Topic Two, Patient Preferences.

1P PEDIATRIC NOTES

Many of the general principles and concepts stated in this topic are as suitable for pediatrics as for medicine. There are, however, significant differences between the medical ethics of adult care and of care for infants and children. We do not review the pediatric issues in depth. We simply call attention to some particular questions where these differences are notable and should be familiar to ethics consultants and ethics committee members. To this Topic of Medical Indications, we append a note regarding decisions to forego interventions for children and regarding determination of death. It is important to remark that the major questions in pediatric ethics are-ssignificantly influenced by the fact that decision making is almost always done by the surrogates rather than the patients, making the Topics "Patient Preferences" (in light of surrogate decisions) and "Quality of Life" particularly important. Fuller treatment of these issues can be found in Frankel LR, Goldworth A, Rorty MV, Silverman WD (Eds.). *Ethical Dilemmas in Pediatrics.* Cambridge: Cambridge University Press; 2005.

1.1P Decisions to Forgo Interventions for Children

With infants and children, as with adults, recommendations must sometimes be made about what forms of care are indicated when death is likely. Although it is often psychologically and emotionally more difficult to accept the death of an infant or child, pediatricians must sometimes recommend that certain interventions are not medically indicated, because they are futile, providing no or, at best, minimal benefits, or because they impose burdens disproportionate to their benefits. All of the cautions about the concept of futility mentioned previously should be observed. Also, certain legal criteria relevant to foregoing treatment for children should be familiar to clinicians and consultants. The statement earlier (Section 1.2.2, Comment) about the use of the word "futility" in discussions with patients and family is even more appropriate when discussing with parents the futility of interventions for their child. Framing the discussion in the principle of proportionality is advisable (see Section 3.3.5).

Cohen R, Kim E. Chapter 2.1: The extremely premature infant at the crossroads; Whitney S. Chapter 2.2: The extremely premature infant at the crossroads: ethical and legal considerations. In: Frankel LB, Goldworth A, Rorty MV, Silverman WA, eds. *Ethical Dilemmas in Pediatrics.* New York, NY: Cambridge University Press; 2005:34–36; 37–51.

1.2P Determination of Death for Children

The clinical method of determining death by brain criteria may be used for infants and children, but special caution is advised, because death cannot be determined with the same degree of certainty in young children as in adults. It is assumed, although not proven, that the child's brain is more resistant to insults leading to death. Physicians responsible for making this determination in children should be familiar with the special clinical issues. In addition to the general criteria (e.g., coma, apnea, absence of brainstem function demonstrated by nonreactive pupils, absence of eye movement, flaccid tone, no spontaneous movement other than spinal cord reflexes, and a ruling-out of hypothermia and hypotension), tests that are only confirmatory in adults are advisable in children, namely, EEG and cerebral blood-flow studies. An observation period of at least 48 hours is recommended between observations.

Naturally, the greatest sympathy and understanding must be extended to parents whose children have died. It is particularly important to make clear that death by brain criteria is distinct from vegetative condition; the term "brain death" confuses the two and should be avoided. Similarly, pediatricians should not speak of "removing life support" when ventilators are supporting breathing after a determination of death by brain criteria. The child is not alive and the ventilator is not supporting life but only physiological functions. Such language only reinforces the mistaken notion that the parents have "let their child die" by authorizing removal of ventilatory support.

Banasiak KJ, Lister G. Brain death in children. *Curr Opin Pediatr.* 2003;15(3):288–299.

Frankel LR, Randle CJ. Chapter 6: Complexities in the management of a brain-dead child; Goldworth A. Chapter 7: The moral arena in the management of a brain-dead child. In: Frankel LR, Goldworth A, Rorty MV, Silverman WA, eds. *Ethical Dilemmas in Pediatrics.* New York, NY: Cambridge University Press; 2005:135–140; 140–147.

Task Force on Brain Death in Children. Guidelines for the determination of brain death in children. *Pediatrics.* 1987;80:298–299.

Patient Preferences

This chapter discusses the second topic that is essential to the analysis of an ethical problem in clinical medicine, namely, the preferences of patients. By *preferences of patients we mean the choices that persons make when they are faced with decisions about health and medical treatment.* These choices reflect the patient's own experience, beliefs, and values as informed by the physician's recommendations. The previous topic, "Medical Indications," concerns the physician's clinical judgment about a patient's medical condition and about interventions that might objectively improve deficits in that condition. When there are medical indications for treatment, a physician should propose a treatment plan that a patient may accept or refuse. We will discuss the following in this chapter: (1) The ethical principle of respect for the autonomy of the patient; (2) the legal, clinical, and psychological significance of patient preferences; (3) informed consent; (4) decisional capacity; (5) truth in medical communication; (6) cultural and religious beliefs; (7) refusal of treatment; (8) advance directives; (9) surrogate decisions; (10) the challenging patient; and (11) alternative medicine.

2.0.1 The Principle of Respect for Autonomy

Respect for autonomy is the guiding ethical principle of the Topic of Patient Preferences. Respect for autonomy is one aspect of a larger principle, namely, respect for persons, which is a fundamental principle of all morality. *Respect for persons affirms that each and every person has moral value and dignity in his or her own right.* In this sense, the principle of respect applies to every encounter between persons, including those between a physician and a patient. *One implication of respect for persons is a respect for personal autonomy, that is, acknowledging the moral right of every individual to choose and follow his or her own plan of life and actions.*

47

In clinical ethics, respect for the autonomy of the patient signifies that physicians' judgments about how to benefit their patients should never ignore or override the preferences of those patients. Patients have the right to freely accept or reject physician's recommendations. Their response to the physician's recommendations should reflect their own values for their own lives. The physician must be confident that medical interventions are acceptable to the patient. As a moral principle, respect for autonomy is a "two-way street": the autonomy of physicians to act only on their best judgment about how best to benefit a patient medically, must also be respected. Therefore, respect for patient autonomy does not imply that patients have the right to demand inappropriate treatment, or that a physician must accede to any and every request of a patient if it conflicts with the physician's best judgment.

While physicians must always respect the autonomy of their patients, in practice, many forces may obstruct and limit the ability of patients to express their preferences. In clincal ethics, respect for patient preferences takes place within a therapeutic relationship, that is, when some health problem prompts a patient to seek help from a physician and a physician responds with diagnosis, advice, and a proposed treatment. In this relationship, physicians possess a de facto power: they have knowledge and skills that the patient needs. Also, patients are often so ill that they cannot clearly formulate or express preferences: they simply want and need help. Therefore, the therapeutic relationship can be distorted by what has been called "physician paternalism": a physician assumes that his or her medical judgment alone should determine the course of care. Modern medical ethics repudiates this sort of paternalism. Instead, both the physician and the patient must form an alliance in which medical recommendations and patient preferences together guide the course of care. This chapter discusses how the ethical principle of respect for autonomy should sustain the therapeutic relationship in general, as well as in those circumstances when preferences are compromised or confused. This chapter examines the conditions for free, informed choice by patients, the strategies that should be employed when the patient is unable to make such a choice, and situations in which a refusal of a physician's recommendation appears to be contrary to the best interests of the patient or causes harm to others. Patient preferences have clinical, legal, and psychological significance.

Beauchamp TL, Childress JF. Respect for autonomy. In: Beauchamp TL, Childress JF, eds. *Principles of Biomedical Ethics*. 6th ed. New York, NY: Oxford University Press; 2009:99–148.

Jennings B. Autonomy. In: Steinbock B, ed. *The Oxford Handbook of Bioethics*. New York, NY: Oxford University Press; 2009:chap 3.

2.0.2 Clinical Significance of Patient Preferences

Attending to patient preferences is essential to good clinical care. Patients who collaborate with their physicians to reach a shared health care decision have greater trust in the doctor-patient relationship, cooperate more fully to implement the shared decision, and express greater satisfaction with their health care. Research has shown that patients with chronic diseases, such as hypertension, non-insulin-dependent diabetes mellitus, peptic ulcer disease, and rheumatoid arthritis, enjoy better health outcomes when they ask questions, express opinions, and make their preferences known.

Similarly, studies show that some physicians are more likely than others to invite the expression of patient preferences and to encourage a participatory decision-making style rather than a controlling style in the therapeutic relationship. A participatory style is associated with primary care training, skill in interviewing that facilitates empathic listening and communication, and the opportunity to spend time with patients. This approach, in which physicians and patients share authority and responsibility in order to build therapeutic alliances, is sometimes referred to as "patient-centered medicine."

Different patients may express different but entirely reasonable preferences when faced with the same medical indications. As medicine has become more effective, a particular problem can often be treated by several medically reasonable options, and each option is associated with different risks and benefits for the patient. For example, to avoid the risk of perioperative death, some patients with lung cancer may choose radiation therapy over surgery despite there being a lower 5-year survival rate with radiation. Similarly, some women may choose prophylactic mastectomy over watchful waiting when told they have a strong genetic propensity to breast cancer; some men may choose watchful waiting over surgery for early cancer of the prostate. Respect for the autonomy of the patient implies that a physician should, after explaining his or her own preferences, honor the patient's preference among medically reasonable options.

It is increasingly common for patients to research their condition on Web sites or to learn about treatment options from the media. This information may enhance understanding and cooperation, but it can also be erroneous or inappropriate for the patient's actual condition. The physician should, to the extent possible, explain this difference to patients. Respect for the patient's autonomy does not require the physician to accede to such preferences if they are medically inappropriate.

2.0.3 Legal Significance of Patient Preferences: Self-Determination

American law recognizes that all persons have a fundamental right to control their own body and the right to be protected from unwanted intrusions. Two classic judicial opinions state this principle succinctly:

Every human being of adult years and of sound mind has a right to determine what shall be done with his body.

Schloendorff v Society of New York Hospital (NY 1914).

Anglo-American law starts with the premise of thoroughgoing self-determination. It follows that each man is considered to be master of his own body, and he may, if he be of sound mind, prohibit the performance of life-saving surgery or other medical treatment.

Natanson v Kline (KS 1960).

All states now have laws requiring informed consent for medical treatment, except in certain emergency situations. The legal requirement of explicit consent for specific treatment protects the legal rights of patients to control what is done to their own bodies. Bodily intrusions without consent constitute an illegal battery. Also, failure to obtain adequate informed consent may also open a physician to a charge of negligence. Finally, apart from clinical skill and carefulness, a respect for patient preferences, good communication, and a participatory style of dealing with patients are known to be the most effective protection that physicians have against malpractice lawsuits. Studies show that patients are much less inclined to bring legal action against physicians who exhibit these behaviors.

2.0.4 Psychological Significance of Patient Preferences: Control

Respect for patient preferences is psychologically significant because the ability to express preferences and have others respect them is crucial to a sense of personal worth. The patient, already threatened by disease, may have a vital need for some sense of control. Indeed, patients and families often struggle to control situations that are beyond human control (see Section 1.2.2.). When patient preferences are ignored or devalued, patients are likely to distrust and perhaps disregard physicians' recommendations. When patients are overtly or covertly uncooperative, the effectiveness of therapy is threatened. Furthermore, patient preferences are important, because their expression may lead to the discovery of other factors, such as fears, fantasies, or unusual beliefs, that the physician should consider in dealing with the patient.

We ask six questions that comprise the issues that must be raised in identifying and assessing an ethical problem regarding patient preferences.

(1) Has the patient been informed of benefits and risks, understood this information, and given consent?
(2) Is the patient mentally capable and legally competent, and is there evidence of incapacity?
(3) If mentally capable, what preferences about treatment is the patient stating?
(4) If incapacitated, has the patient expressed prior preferences?
(5) Who is the appropriate surrogate to make decisions for the incapacitated patient?
(6) Is the patient unwilling or unable to cooperate with medical treatment? If so, why?

2.1 INFORMED CONSENT

Informed consent is the practical application of respect for the patient's autonomy. When patients consult a physician for a suspected medical problem, they usually state the problem as they see it. They then request help, either explicitly or implicitly. Physicians make a diagnosis and recommend treatment.

2.1.1 Question One—Has the Patient been Informed of Benefits and Risks, Understood This Information, and Given Consent?

In the process called "Informed Consent," physicians explain their opinion about the nature of the patient's problem, recommend a course of treatment, give the reasons for the recommendation, propose options for alternative treatments, and explain the benefits and risks of all options. The patient, ideally, understands the information, assesses the treatment choices, and agrees (or disagrees) to accept the physician's recommendation.

Informed consent constitutes a central feature of an encounter between physicians and patients, characterized by mutual participation, good communication, mutual respect, and shared decision making. Informed consent requires a dialogue between physician and patient leading to agreement about the course of medical care. Informed consent establishes a reciprocal relationship between physician and patient. After initial consent to treatment has occurred, an ongoing dialogue between patient and physician, concerning the patient's continuing medical needs, reinforces the original consent. A properly negotiated informed consent benefits both the physician and the patient—a therapeutic alliance is forged in which the physician's work is facilitated because the patient has realistic expectations about results of the treatment, is prepared for possible complications, and is more likely to be a willing collaborator in the treatment. Despite a vast literature in law and ethics about the importance of informed consent, many studies reveal that physicians are often deficient in observing the practice and the spirit of informed consent.

Law has long required explicit consent to surgery, a serious and possible lethal invasion of the human body. However, consent for medical treatment was usually considered presumed by the very presence of the patient in need. However, the more elaborate practice of informed consent, described earlier, has become ethically and legally vital, as more of medical and surgical care involves lengthy, perhaps lifelong, modifications of personal life. Chemotherapy for many disease conditions lasts for life; organ and tissue transplantation requires continual immunosuppression and surveillance. The care of all chronic diseases necessarily requires the understanding, acceptance, and cooperation of patients. These features of modern medicine may make informed consent as much a personal acceptance of changes in one's quality of life as it is permission for a procedure.

Beauchamp TL, Childress JF. The meaning and justification of informed consent. In: Beauchamp TL, Childress JF, eds. *Principles of Biomedical Ethics*. 6th ed. New York, NY: Oxford University Press; 2009:117–134.

Berg JW, Appelbaum PS, Lidz CW, et al. *Informed Consent: Legal Theory and Clinical Practice*. New York, NY: Oxford University Press; 2001.

Lo B. Informed consent. In: Lo B, ed. *Resolving Ethical Dilemmas*. 3rd ed. Philadelphia, PA: Lippincott Williams & Wilkins; 2005:17–27.

Williams J. Consent. In: Singer PA, Viens AM, eds. *The Cambridge Textbook of Bioethics*. New York, NY: Cambridge University Press; 2008: 11–16.

CASE I. Mr. Cure, the patient with pneumococcal meningitis, is told that he needs immediate antibiotic therapy. After he is informed of the nature of his disease, the benefits and burdens of treatment, and the possible consequences of nontreatment, he expresses his preference by consenting to the antibiotic therapy. A therapeutic alliance that is clinically, ethically, and emotionally satisfactory is formed and reinforced when the patient recovers.

CASE II. Ms. Cope is a 42-year-old woman who was diagnosed as having insulin-dependent diabetes at the age of 18. Insulin was prescribed and a dietary regimen recommended. In the intervening years, she has complied with her dietary and medical regimen but has experienced repeated episodes of ketoacidosis and hypoglycemia. Her physician has regularly discussed with Ms. Cope the course of her disease and the treatment plan and has inquired about her difficulties in managing her condition. The physician proposes that Ms. Cope consider an implantable insulin pump that could improve glycemic control.

COMMENT. Case I exemplifies what might be called routine consent. The physician expresses clinical judgment by making recommendations to the patient regarding an appropriate course of care. The patient makes known his preference by consulting the physician for diagnosis and treatment and by accepting the physician's recommendations. Case II is also an example of routine consent, but it occurs in a chronic disease setting. Ms. Cope's doctor was assiduous in informing and educating her patient. Ms. Cope accepted the treatment regimen, and her compliance with it shows her preferences. She is now considering whether she will accept the benefits and risk of the insulin pump. Patients with chronic diseases, which often have variable courses far into the future, must consider a wider range of consequences. We shall see problems develop in both these cases in the following pages.

2.1.2 Definition and Standards of Disclosure

Informed consent is defined as the willing acceptance of a medical intervention by a patient after adequate disclosure by the physician of the nature of the intervention, its risks and benefits, and also its alternatives with their risks and benefits. How should the adequacy of disclosure of information by a physician be determined? One approach is to ask what a reasonable and prudent physician would tell a patient. This approach, which was the legal standard in some of the early informed consent cases, is increasingly being replaced by a new standard, namely, what information do reasonable patients need to know to make reasonable decisions. The former standard affords greater discretion to the physician; the latter "reasonable patient" is more patient centered. A third standard, sometimes called a "subjective" standard, is patient specific. Under this standard, the information provided is specifically tailored to a particular patient's need for information and understanding. Although the law usually requires that the physician meet only the reasonable-patient standard, a physician who engages in a participatory style of shared decision-making should aspire to the requirements of a subjective standard.

2.1.3 Scope of Disclosure

Many studies show that patients desire more information from their physicians; many practitioners are aware that their patients appreciate information. In recent years, candid disclosure has become the norm. *It is widely agreed that disclosure should include (1) the patient's current medical status, including the likely course if no treatment is provided; (2) the interventions that might improve prognosis, including a description and the risks and benefits of those procedures and some estimation of probabilities and uncertainties associated with the interventions; (3) a professional opinion about alternatives open to the patient; and (4) a recommendation that is made on the basis of the physician's best clinical judgment.*

In conveying this information, physicians should avoid technical terms, attempt to translate statistical data into everyday probabilities, ask whether the patient understands the information, and invite questions. Physicians are not obliged, as one court said, to give each patient "a mini-medical education." Still, physicians should strive to educate their patients about their specific medical needs and options.

As we mentioned in Section 2.0.2, physicians are not the only sources of medical information: media, Web sites, advocacy organizations, and many other sources provide information of various quality. Persons often come to the physician with files full of articles. It falls to the physician to interpret this information and, above all, to evaluate its relevance to this particular patient.

There is ethical debate about whether the scope of disclosure should include information about the experience of the physician, for example, disclosing the number of previous procedures performed with the data being physician specific rather than national, outcome data. While physicians routinely refer patients to specialists for problems and procedures in which they are not expert, they may not be comfortable telling a patient about the extent of their experience with a procedure they are about to perform. Some physicians learn a technique in a weekend course and perform it in their offices on Monday. It is our opinion that it is ethically appropriate to disclose levels of experience, and it is obligatory to do so in situations where the procedure is necessary but has significant risks or is elective. The patient is then able to make an informed choice about how to proceed.

The moral and legal obligations of disclosure vary with the situation; they become more stringent as the treatment situation moves from emergency through elective to experimental. In some emergency situations, very little information need be provided. Any attempt to inform may cost precious time. Ethically and legally, information can be curtailed in emergencies (see Section 2.4.3). For nonemergency or elective treatments, much more information should be provided. Finally, fully detailed and thorough information should accompany any experimental or innovative treatment.

D'Agincourt-Canning L, Johnston C. Disclosure. In: Singer PA, Viens AM, eds. *The Cambridge Textbook of Bioethics*. New York, NY: Cambridge University Press; 2008:24–30.

2.1.4 Comprehension

Discussions of informed consent usually emphasize the amount and kind of information the doctor should provide. The patient's comprehension is equally as important as the adequacy of the information. Many studies suggest that comprehension by patients of medical information is limited and inadequate. Information is often provided in settings and at times when the patient is distressed or distracted. At the same time, studies suggest that communication is often poorly accomplished and that little effort is made to overcome barriers to comprehension. The physician has an ethical obligation to make reasonable efforts to ensure comprehension. Explanations should be given clearly and simply; questions should be asked to assess understanding. Written instructions or printed materials should be provided. Video or computer programs should be provided to guide patients who face complicated decisions, such as choosing between options for treatment of breast cancer or prostate cancer. Educational programs for patients with chronic disease should be arranged. While physicians have the primary responsibility to inform their patients, other clinicians, particularly nurses, may supplement and enhance the information provided by the physician.

2.1.5 Documentation of Consent

The process of informed consent is documented in a signed consent form that is entered in the patient's record. Health care institutions require signed documentation before certain medical and most surgical or invasive diagnostic procedures are initiated. The document typically names the procedure and states that the risks and benefits have been explained to the patient. It is sometimes believed—wrongly—that a signed consent form is legal proof that a patient has given consent. In fact, the signed consent form in the absence of a consent discussion does not prove that the necessary discussion leading to an informed consent has taken place. The actual process and details of the consent interview should be documented by the physician in the medical record. The signed consent form is not a substitute for this more complete documentation.

2.1.6 Difficulties With Informed Consent

Many studies reveal that physicians often fail to conduct ethically and legally satisfactory consent negotiations. Physicians may be trapped in technical language, troubled by the uncertainty intrinsic to all medical information, worried about alarming the patient, or hurried and pressed by multiple duties. In addition, patients may have limited understanding, may be inattentive and distracted, or overcome by fear and anxiety. Selective hearing because of denial, fear, or preoccupation with illness may account for failure to comprehend what one might otherwise understand. Patients may believe that decisions are the physician's prerogative; physicians may not appreciate the rationale for the patient's participation.

These inadequacies in the informed consent process may be due to a belief by some physicians that the informed consent requirement imposes an undesirable and perhaps impossible task: undesirable because adequately informing a patient takes too much time and might create unnecessary anxiety, and impossible because no medically uneducated and clinically inexperienced patient can truly grasp the significance of the information the physician must disclose. For these reasons, physicians sometimes dismiss the informed consent requirement as a bureaucratically necessary ritual. This is a sadly limited view of the ethical purpose of informed consent. Informed consent is not merely pushing information at a patient. It is an opportunity to initiate a dialogue between physicians and their patients in which both attempt to arrive at a mutually satisfactory course of action.

Informed consent should result in shared decision making. The process, while difficult, is not impossible and is always open to improvement.

2.1.7 Truthful Communication

Communications between physicians and patients should be truthful; that is, statements should be in accord with facts. If the facts are uncertain, that uncertainty should be acknowledged. Deception, by stating what is untrue or by omitting what is true, should be avoided. These ethical principles should govern all human communication. However, in the communication between patients and physicians, certain ethical problems about truthfulness may emerge. Does the patient really want to know the truth? What if the truth, once known, causes harm? Might not deception help by supporting hope? Traditionally, medical ethics has given ambiguous answers to these questions: while some past authors favored truthfulness, others recommended beneficent deception. More recently, with the prominence of the doctrine of informed consent, truthfulness has been commended as the ethical course of action.

Beauchamp TL, Childress JF. Veracity. In: Beauchamp TL, Childress JF, eds. *Principles of Biomedical Ethics*. 6th ed. New York, NY: Oxford University Press; 2009:288–295.

Hebert PC, Hoffmaster B, Glass KC. Truth telling. In: Singer PA, Viens AM, eds. *The Cambridge Textbook of Bioethics*. New York, NY: Cambridge University Press; 2008:36–42.

Lo B. Avoiding deception and nondisclosure. In: Lo B, ed. *Resolving Ethical Dilemmas: A Guide for Clinicians*. 3rd ed. Philadelphia, PA: Lippincott Williams & Wilkins; 2005:45–53.

CASE I. Mr. R.S., a 65-year-old man, comes to his physician with complaints of weight loss and mild abdominal discomfort. The patient, whom the physician knows well, has just retired from a busy career and has made plans for a round-the-world tour with his wife. Studies reveal mild elevation in liver function tests and a questionable mass in the tail of the pancreas. At the beginning of his interview with his physician to discuss the test results, Mr. R.S. remarks, "Doc, I hope you don't have any bad news for me. We've got big plans." Ordinarily, a procedure to obtain tissue to confirm pancreatic cancer would be the next step. The physician wonders whether he should put this off until Mr. R.S. returns from his trip. Should the physician's opinion that Mr. R.S. may have pancreatic cancer be revealed to him at this time?

COMMENT. Contemporary bioethics strongly affirms the patient's right to the truth. The arguments in support of this position are:

1. General ethical arguments favor a strong moral duty to tell the truth as contributory to personal relationships and social cohesion. This general obligation is not easily overridden by speculative possible harms that might come from knowing the truth.
2. Suspicion on the part of the physician that truthful disclosure would be harmful to the patient may be founded on little or no evidence. It may arise more from the physician's own uneasiness at being a "bearer of bad news" than from the patient's inability to accept the information.
3. Patients have a need for the truth if they are to make rational decisions about actions and plans for life.
4. Concealment of the truth is likely to undermine the patient–physician relationship. In case of serious illness, it is particularly important that this relationship be strong.
5. Toleration of concealment by the physician may undermine the trust that the public should have in the profession. Widespread belief that physicians are not truthful would create an atmosphere in which persons who fear being deceived would not seek needed care.
6. Recent studies have shown that most patients with diagnoses of serious illness wish to know their diagnosis. Similarly, recent studies are unable to document harmful effects of full disclosure.

RECOMMENDATION. Mr. R.S. should be told the truth. He probably has cancer of the pancreas and should have a procedure to obtain tissue for pathological analysis. The considerations in favor of truthful disclosure, in our opinion, establish a strong ethical obligation on the physician to tell the truth to patients about their diagnosis and its treatment. The following considerations are relevant:

(a) Speaking truthfully means relating the facts of the situation. This should be done in a manner measured to perceptions of the hearer's emotional resilience and intellectual comprehension. The truth may be brutal, but the telling of it should not be. A measured and sensitive disclosure is demanded by respect for the patient's autonomy. It reinforces the patient's ability to deliberate and choose; it does not overwhelm this ability. It is advisable to open such a conversation with a question about how much detail the patient wishes to know and whether the patient may wish some other person to be informed.

(b) Truthful disclosure has implications for Mr. R.S.'s plans. Further diagnostic studies might be done and appropriate treatments chosen. The trip might be delayed or canceled. Estate and advance care planning might be considered. Mr. R.S. should have the opportunity to reflect on these matters and to take control of his future.

CASE II. Mr. S.P., a 55-year-old teacher, has had chest pains and several fainting spells during the past 3 months. He reluctantly visits a physician at his wife's urging. He is very nervous and anxious and says to the physician at the beginning of the interview that he abhors doctors and hospitals. On physical examination, he has classic signs of tight aortic stenosis, confirmed by echocardiogram. The physician wants to recommend cardiac catheterization and probably cardiac surgery. However, given his impression of this patient, he is worried that full disclosure of the risks of catheterization would lead the patient to refuse the procedure.

COMMENT. In this case, the anticipated harm is much more specific and dangerous than the harm contemplated in Case I. Hesitation about revealing the risks of a diagnostic or therapeutic procedure is based on the fear the patient will make a judgment detrimental to health and life. Also, in this case there is better reason to suspect this patient will react badly to the information than will the patient in Case I.

RECOMMENDATION. The arguments in favor of truthful disclosure apply equally to this case and to Case I. Whether or not catheterization is accepted, the patient will need further medical care. In fact, the situation is urgent. This patient needs, above all, the benefits of a good and trusting relationship with a competent physician. Honesty is more likely to create that relationship than deception. Also, the physician's fears about the patient's refusal may be exaggerated. The physician might also be concerned about the family's reaction if Mr. S.P. died unexpectedly during catheterization. Although Mr. S.P. has avoided physicians in the past, now that he is seriously ill, he may become more accepting of the help that medicine can offer. The physician would be at serious fault if the patient died without having had the opportunity to consider the options for care.

2.1.8 Placebo Treatment

Placebo treatment is a clinical intervention intended by the physician to benefit the patient, not by any known physiological mechanism of the intervention, but because of certain psychological or psychophysical effects due to the positive expectations, beliefs, and hopes of the patient. The intervention might be, as it was often in the past, an inert substance, a sugar pill, or, as it is frequently practiced today, vitamin pills, over-the-counter analgesics, or saline injections. That such interventions do result in a *placebo effect*, such as relief of pain, has long been demonstrated. Recent studies reveal that almost half of American physicians utilize placebo treatments on a regular basis.

Tilburt, JC, Emanuel E, et al. Prescribing "placebo treatments": results of a national survey of US internists and rheumatologists. *BMJ*. 2008;337:1938.

Placebo treatment raises a problem of truth telling, because it seems inevitably to involve deception. The physician knows that the intervention does not have the objective properties necessary for efficacy and the patient is kept ignorant of this fact. In some cases, the deception is an outright moral offense, motivated solely by the desire to charge the patient for a procedure or to "get the patient off my back"; in other cases, placebo deception may be motivated by the judgment that a harmless intervention may achieve a positive result. This raises a genuine ethical question: the duty not to deceive seems to conflict with the duty to benefit without doing harm.

Placebo agents are now commonly used in controlled clinical trials of therapy for non–life-threatening conditions. However, no deception is involved, because research subjects must be informed that they will be randomized and may receive either an active drug or an inert substance. This practice is certainly ethical. At present, there is a broad consensus among ethicists that clinical use of placebos is unethical.

Beauchamp TL, Childress JF. Intentional nondisclosure. In: Beauchamp TL, Childress JF, eds. *Principles of Biomedical Ethics*. 6th ed. New York, NY: Oxford University Press; 2009:124–127.

Brody H. The lie that heals: the ethics of giving placebos. *Ann Intern Med*. 1982;97:112–118.

CASE I. A 73-year-old widow lives with her son. He brings her to a physician because she has become extremely lethargic and often confused. The physician determines that, after being widowed 2 years earlier, she had difficulty sleeping, had been prescribed hypnotics, and is now physically dependent on them. The physician determines the best course would be to withdraw her from her present medication by a trial on placebos.

CASE II. A 62-year-old man has had a total proctocolectomy and ileostomy for colon cancer. Evidence of any remaining tumor is absent, the wound is healing well, and the ileostomy is functioning. On the eighth day after surgery, he complains of crampy abdominal pain and requests medication. The physician first prescribes antispasmodic drugs, but the patient's complaints persist. The patient requests morphine, which had relieved his postoperative pain. The physician is reluctant to prescribe opiates because repeated studies suggest that the pain is psychological, and the physician knows that opiates will cause constipation. She contemplates a trial of placebo.

COMMENT. Any situation in which placebo use involves deliberate deception should be viewed as ethically suspect. The strong moral obligations of truthfulness and honesty prohibit deception; the danger to the patient–physician relationship advises against it. Any exception to this strict obligation would have to fulfill the following conditions: (1) The condition to be treated should be known as one that has high response rates to placebo, for example, mild mental depression or postoperative pain; (2) the alternative to placebo is either continued illness or the use of a drug with known toxicity and addictability, for example, hypnotics as in Case I or opioids in Case II; (3) the patient wishes to be treated and cured, if possible; and (4) the patient insists on a prescription.

RECOMMENDATION. The use of a placebo in Case I is not justified. The patient is not demanding medication. The problem of addiction should be confronted directly. There will be ample opportunity to develop a good relationship with this patient. Subsequent discovery of deception might undermine this relationship. Use of placebo in Case II is tempting but not ethically justifiable. In favor of placebo use, the patient is demanding relief. Morphine has adverse side effects. A short trial of placebo may be effective in relieving pain and avoiding the harm associated with opioids. However, explanation may be as effective as placebo use. The deceptive placebo can destroy the trust that creates the important and therapeutic placebo effect and can undermine the patient's confidence in the physician. A participatory style of decision-making is based on honest communication. It may be possible, for example, to perform a "mini-experiment" with the patient's consent: explain that two forms of pills will be offered, one active, the other inert, and the patient will blindly choose which one to take. Consultation with the hospital Pain Service is recommended.

2.1.9 Completeness of Disclosure

Disclosure of options for treatment of a patient's condition should be complete, that is, containing all information that a thoughtful person would need to make a good decision in their own behalf. It should include the options that the physician recommends. It should also include other options that the physician may believe are less desirable but which are still medically reasonable. In so doing, physicians may make it clear why they consider these other options less desirable.

D'Agincourt-Canning L, Johnston C. Disclosure. In: Singer PA, Viens AM, eds. *The Cambridge Textbook of Bioethics.* New York, NY: Cambridge University Press. 2008:24–30.

CASE I. A 41-year-old woman has a breast biopsy that reveals cancer. The physician knows that this patient has a history of noncompliance and cancellation of medical appointments. In light of this, the physician believes that the best treatment approach would be a modified radical mastectomy; this treatment would require less continued care than a lumpectomy and 5 weeks of outpatient radiotherapy. Should the physician omit mention of this second option because she is concerned that after a lumpectomy, the patient may not keep her radiotherapy appointments?

RECOMMENDATION. The entire range of options should be explained with a careful delineation of the risks and benefits of each. Making a strong argument in favor of the option the physician considers best is ethically appropriate. However, the patient should be left free to choose, even if the physician believes she may choose the less effective option. Coercion and manipulation of the patient should be carefully avoided. Ultimately, the patient must make decisions about breast surgery and keeping appointments. The physician must provide the patient with information and encourage her to complete whatever form of treatment she elects to receive.

COMMENT. The dialogue between physicians and patients is not only inhibited by limitations of physician communication and patient comprehension, it is also limited by the failure of many physicians to listen carefully to their patients' words and the emotions underlying them. Finally, the time limits for patient visits imposed by some managed care plans and clinics, and reimbursement policies that compensate for procedures but not for education, discourage good communication. The importance of improved communication between doctors and patients should be obvious in this age of information.

2.1.10 Refusal of Information

Persons have a right to information about themselves. Similarly, they have the right to refuse information or to ask the physician not to inform them.

CASE I. Mr. A.J. is scheduled for surgery for spinal stenosis. The neurosurgeon begins to discuss the risks and benefits of this surgery. The patient responds, "Doctor I don't want to hear anything more. I want the surgery. I realize there are risks, and I have confidence in you." The surgeon is concerned that he has not completed an adequate disclosure.

CASE II. Mrs. Care, with MS, had shown little interest during the early years of her illness in learning about the possible course of her disease. She refused frequent offers by the physician to discuss it. However, on one of her repeated admissions for treatment of urinary tract infection, she states that, had she known what life would be like, she would have refused permission for treatment of other life-threatening problems. The patient's mental status is difficult to evaluate. Her doctor thinks she is severely depressed; the intensivist believes she shows signs of early dementia. Should she have been informed of her prognosis at an earlier time even though unwilling to engage in such discussions with her physician?

RECOMMENDATION. In Case I, Mr. A.J.'s refusal of information should be respected. His surgeon has no obligation to press the matter, although he may repeat the offer of information at appropriate times. The surgeon must make a full notation in the chart that the patient has refused information. It is desirable to seek the patient's permission to discuss the detail of the procedure with an involved family member. If and when patients desire additional information, clinicians should be prepared to offer it.

Case II poses a difficult case. Here we opt for more rather than less disclosure, because the condition, though untreatable, is long lasting. The patient's long-term autonomy is respected more by providing as much information as possible to enable her to make more choices while she is physically and mentally able to learn coping mechanisms in advance. Although it might be tempting to withhold information to protect the patient, a better alternative would be to give the patient general information sufficient to indicate the seriousness of her condition as well as the uncertainty about the time, the severity, and the extent of the problems that MS can cause. This avoids the extremes of withholding too much too long or disclosing too much too soon. Considerable tact is required to find the proper balance of disclosure and reticence. Furthermore, the disclosures made as the condition worsens must be adjusted in the light of the impairments to the patient's capacity. In some cases of late-stage MS an associated dementia appears. It would be advisable to make disclosures before the patient's capacity is so severely impaired that she cannot understand.

Lo B. Refusal of treatment by competent, informed patients. In: Lo B, ed. *Resolving Ethical Dilemmas. A Guide for Clinicians.* 4th ed. Philadelphia, PA: Lippincott Williams & Wilkins; 2009:83–87.

2.1.11 *Disclosure of Medical Error*

When medical errors, as defined in Section 1.4, occur, what obligation does the physician and the hospital have to disclose errors to patients? Some errors are due to negligence, but the majority are due to accident, misinformation, or organizational malfunction. Some errors do not cause harm; others effect serious harm. When medical errors occur, what obligations do physicians have to disclose them?

CASE. The patient described in Section 2.1.9 is treated by modified radical mastectomy and reconstructive breast surgery. Postoperatively, she develops persistent swelling and drainage of the breast and a fever consistent with a breast abscess. She is returned to the operating room for exploration of the operative site. The surgeon discovers that a sponge had been left in the surgical wound. It is removed, and the abscess is treated. The patient recovered and was discharged. Should the physician inform the patient that a mistake had been made?

RECOMMENDATION. Disclosure is required because harm was done to this patient by the medical error. Although the outcome was satisfactory, the patient required a second operation with attendant risks; her hospital stay, with its attendant risks, was prolonged; chemotherapy was delayed, and costs were incurred. A fundamental duty of respect for persons dictates that apology be offered the patient for harms of this sort. The surgeon should inform and apologize to the patient and report the error to the hospital, which should also apologize. Appropriate compensation should be provided.

COMMENT. Any inclination to hide medical mistakes must be discouraged. Secrecy is unethical and may be counterproductive. Mistakes must be reported for risk management and quality assurance purposes, and organizations should have procedures for reporting and correcting and preventing errors. Charges should be waived and appropriate compensation provided; settlement of financial claims, even without suit, may be considered. A climate of disclosure and honesty is necessary to maintain patient confidence and trust in the relationship with their physicians and with the health care institutions. Malpractice actions are certainly possible, particularly if the error is the result of negligence, but threat of legal claims is reduced in a climate of confidence and honesty. Errors that are truly harmless, without any adverse effects for the patient (e.g., an incorrect dosage of medication is prepared, but corrected before administration), must be reported within the system for control purposes. Although it is not obligatory to disclose harmless error, it is advisable to do so to sustain the climate of honesty in the relationship between the patient and physician (see Section 4.11).

Lo B. Disclosing errors. In: Lo B, ed. *Resolving Ethical Dilemmas. A Guide for Clinicians.* 4th ed. Philadelphia, PA: Lippincott Williams & Wilkins; 2009:243–250.

2.2 DECISIONAL CAPACITY

Informed consent and truthful disclosure presuppose that the patient possesses the legal competence and mental capacity to hear and comprehend communication. There are many situations in clinical care in which patients appear to, or obviously do, lack this capacity.

2.2.1 Question Two—Is the Patient Mentally Capable and Legally Competent, and Is There Evidence of Incapacity?

Consent to treatment is complicated because some patients lack the mental capacity to understand information or to make choices. In the law, the terms *competence* and *incompetence* indicate whether persons have the legal authority to affect certain personal choices, such as managing their finances or making health care decisions. Judges alone have the right to rule that a person is legally incompetent and to issue a court order or appoint a guardian. In medical care, however, persons who are legally competent may have their mental capacities compromised by illness, anxiety, and/or pain. We refer to this clinical situation as *decisional capacity* or *incapacity* to distinguish it from the legal determination of competency. It is necessary to assess decisional capacity as an essential part of the informed consent process.

Beauchamp TL, Childress JF. Capacity for autonomous choice. In: Beauchamp TL, Childress JF, eds. *Principles of Biomedical Ethics*. 6th ed. New York, NY: Oxford University Press; 2009:111–117.

Chalmers J. Capacity. In: Singer PA, Viens AM, eds. *The Cambridge Textbook of Bioethics*. New York, NY: Cambridge University Press; 2008:17–23.

Grisso T, Appelbaum P. *Assessing Competence to Consent to Treatment*. New York, NY: Oxford University Press; 1998.

Lo B. Decision-making capacity. In: Lo B, ed. *Resolving Ethical Dilemmas. A Guide for Clinicians*. 4th ed. Philadelphia, PA: Lippincott Williams & Wilkins; 2009:75–82.

2.2.2 Definition of Decisional Capacity

In a medical setting, a patient's capacity to consent to or refuse care requires the ability to understand relevant information, to appreciate the medical situation and its possible consequences, to communicate a choice, and to engage in rational deliberation about one's own values in relation to the physician's recommendations about treatment options. Patients who obviously possess these abilities may make decisions about their care and their right to do so should be respected. Patients, who clearly lack these abilities because, for example, they are comatose, unconscious, or are disoriented and delusional, are unable to make informed, reasonable choices. For them, a surrogate decision-maker is required. However, many patients fall between these two situations: their decisional capacity may be questionable. Many ethical cases involve very sick patients whose mental status may be altered by trauma, fear, pain, physiological imbalance (e.g., hypotension, fever, mental status changes), or from drugs used to treat their medical condition. It is often unclear whether such patients are able to make informed, reasonable decisions for their own welfare.

2.2.3 Determining Decisional Capacity

Decisional capacity refers to the specific acts of comprehending, evaluating, and choosing among realistic options. Determining decisional capacity is a clinical judgment. The first step in making a determination of capacity is to engage the patient in conversation, to observe the patient's behavior, and to talk with third parties—family, friends, or staff. Experienced clinicians will often assess decisional capacity through a simple conversation with the patient, noting inconsistencies, incoherence, and confusion. This sort of evaluation may result in diagnoses such as dementia, delirium, or encephalopathy. However, it is often difficult to discern the signs of mental incapacity. For example, paranoid patients appear normal until certain situations trigger a delusional belief system. Often, unusual decisions may prompt suspicion about mental incapacity: for example, a patient refuses a low-risk, high-benefit treatment without which he or she faces serious injury.

Psychiatric diagnoses such as schizophrenia, depression, or dementia do not, in themselves, rule out the possibility that a patient has mental capacity to make particular decisions. Many persons with mental disease retain the ability to make reasonable decisions about particular medical choices that face them. Rather, the question is how these general psychological states and psychiatric diagnoses actually inhibit the patient's ability to understand and choose in a particular situation. When a clinician doubts a patient's decisional capacity to make particular choices, tests for cognitive functioning, psychiatric disorders, or organic conditions that may affect decisional capacity can be used. The MacArthur Competence Assessment Tool (MacCAT-T) is a commonly used clinical assessment tool. However, no single test is sufficient to capture the complex concept of decisional capacity in a clinical setting. Some conditions, such as an affective state of anxiety or depression, may be transitory or reversible with psychiatric intervention. Other conditions, such as medication-induced confusion, may be resolved by titrating medication properly. But some problems, such as inability to understand simple explanations of facts, or fixed delusions, may be impossible to remedy. The clinical techniques for making an assessment of capacity can be learned by all clinicians, and can be utilized by any trained clinician, including clinical ethicists. In some circumstances, the evidence for incapacity is more complex or obscure, particularly when psychiatric disorders may be present. In such cases, the consultation should be sought from more expert clinicians, such as psychiatrists and clinical psychologists. Also, local law and policy may require assessment by a mental health professional, particularly if guardianship proceedings are contemplated. When clinical evidence is sufficient to show that a patient is decisionally incapacitated, an appropriate surrogate decision-maker assumes authority, as explained in Section 2.4.

Appelbaum P, Grisso T. Assessing patient's capacities to consent to treatment. *N Engl J Med.* 1988;319:1635–1638.

Grisso T, Appelbaum P. *MacArthur Competence Assessment Tool for Treatment.* Sarasota, FL: Professional Resource Press; 2001.

2.2.4 Evaluating Decisional Capacity in Relation to the Need for Intervention: The Sliding Scale Criterion

Usually a patient's capacity is not seriously questioned unless the patient decides to refuse or discontinue medically indicated treatment. When patients reject recommended treatment, clinicians may suspect that the patients' choices may be harmful to their health and welfare. They assume that persons ordinarily do not act contrary to their best interests. *It has been suggested that the stringency of criteria for capacity should vary with the seriousness of the disease and urgency for treatment.* For example, a patient might need to meet only a low standard of capacity to consent to a procedure with substantial, highly probable benefits and minimal, low-probability risk, such as antibiotics for bacterial meningitis. If, however, a patient refuses such an intervention, it must be quite clear that the person understands and freely accepts the risks and dangers of refusing and decides what he or she is about to do. Likewise, greater decisional capacity is necessary to consent to an intervention that poses high risks and offers little benefit. Although this sliding scale stringency test has been criticized as inadequately protecting a patient's right to refuse, it can be helpful to the clinician in deciding whether the refusal should be simply accepted or whether to take further steps to investigate and even take action to counteract the refusal by legal means.

CASE I. Mrs. Cope, the 42-year-old woman with insulin-dependent diabetes, is brought by her husband to the emergency department. She is stuporous, with severe diabetic ketoacidosis and pneumonia. Physicians prescribe insulin and fluids for the ketoacidosis and antibiotics for the pneumonia. Although Mrs. Cope was generally somnolent, she awoke while the IV was being inserted and stated loudly: "Leave me alone. No needles and no hospital. I'm OK." Her husband urged the medical team to disregard the patient's statements, saying, "She is not herself."

COMMENT. We agree with Mr. Cope's assessment of the situation. Mrs. Cope has an acute crisis (ketoacidosis and pneumonia) superimposed on a chronic disease (Type I Diabetes) and she demonstrates progressive stupor during a 2-day period. At this time, she clearly lacks decisional capacity, although she could make decisions 2 days prior to the onset of her illness, and she could possibly make her own decisions again when she recovers from the ketoacidosis, probably within the next 24 hours. At this moment, it would be unethical to be guided by the demands of a stuporous individual who lacks decision-making capacity. The cause of her mental incapacity is known and is reversible. Physicians and surrogate concur on the patient's incapacity and are agreed on the course of treatment in accordance with the patient's best interest. The physicians would be correct to be guided by the wishes of the patient's surrogate, her husband, and to treat Mrs. Cope over her objections. Issues associated with surrogate decision-making are discussed in Section 2.4.

CASE II. In the case presented at Sections 1.0.8 and 2.1.1, Mr. Cure has symptoms and clinical findings diagnostic of bacterial meningitis. He is informed that he needs immediate hospitalization and administration of antibiotics. Although drowsy, he appears to understand the physician's explanation. He refuses treatment and says he wants to go home. The physician explains the extreme dangers of going untreated and the minimal risks of treatment. The young man persists in his refusal.

COMMENT. The physician might presume altered mental status because of fever or metabolic disturbance or brain infection due to meningoencephalitis. However, the patient appears to understand his situation and the consequences of refusal of treatment. Physicians sometimes assume that anyone who refuses a physician's recommendation of necessary or useful treatment must be mentally incapacitated. Refusal of treatment should not, in and of itself, be considered a sign of incapacity. In this case, the clinician's presumption of altered mental status is reinforced by an inexplicable and unexplained refusal of care, with drastic consequences. Is it ethically permissible to treat against his will a patient who is making an irrevocable choice that will result in his death or permanent disability, who gives no reason for this decision, and for whom a clear determination of mental incapacity cannot be made?

In this case, the initial consent for diagnosis was implicit in the young man allowing himself to be brought to the emergency department. Further, he consented to diagnostic procedures, including a spinal fluid examination. The patient's refusal of treatment, however, unexpectedly introduced an incongruity between medical indications and patient preferences. It might be argued that the physician should simply permit the patient to refuse treatment and suffer the consequences, because the patient did not show clear signs of incapacitation or of serious psychiatric impairment and because competent patients have the right to make their own (sometimes risky) decisions. It might also be argued that the clinical status of the patient, a brain infection with fever, justifies a presumption of incapacitation. Certainly, in such a puzzling case, it is ethically obligatory for the physician to probe further to determine why the patient inexplicably refused treatment. Despite the physician's best efforts to explain, has the patient failed to understand and appreciate the nature of the condition or the benefits and risks of treatment and nontreatment? If the patient seems to understand the explanation, is he in denial that he is really ill? Is the patient acting on the basis of some unexpressed fear, mistaken belief, or irrational desire? Through further discussion with the patient, some of these questions might be answered.

Assume, however, that after the most thorough investigation possible under the urgent circumstances, there is no evidence that the patient fails to understand and nothing emerges to suggest denial, fear, mistake, or irrational belief. Should the patient's refusal be respected? Because the medical condition is so serious, should treatment proceed even against the patient's will? This case poses a genuine ethical conflict between the patient's personal autonomy and the physician's duty to impose paternalistic values that favor medical intervention for the patient's own good. A clinical decision to treat the patient or release him must be made quickly. Good ethical reasons can be given for either alternative.

RECOMMENDATION. This patient should be treated despite his refusal. His refusal is enigmatic, insofar as he offers no reason for refusing. Certainly, the clinician should suspect an altered mental status due to high fever and brain infection, but this patient is oriented to time and place, communicates articulately, and appears to understand the consequences of his refusal. There is no time for a thorough psychiatric examination. Given the enigmatic nature of his refusal and the urgent, serious need for treatment, the patient should be treated with antibiotics, even against his will. Should there be time, legal authorization should be sought.

This is a genuine moral dilemma: the principle of beneficence and the principle of autonomy seem to dictate contradictory courses of action. In medical care, dilemmas cannot merely be contemplated; they must be resolved. It is difficult to believe that this young man wishes to die or become permanently damaged neurologically. The conscientious physician faces two evils: to honor a refusal that might not represent the patient's true preferences, leading to the patient's serious disability or death, or to override the refusal in the hope that, subsequently, the patient will recognize the benefit or later realize that his decisional capacity was impaired.

In such situations of moral tension, clinicians may ask themselves five questions that may clarify which course is more ethically acceptable: (1) Did I explain the critical situation in a clear, understandable way? (2) Is it possible that language barriers, education level, or hearing deficits hinder the patient's understanding? (3) Might fear, pain, or lack of trust impair the patient's understanding? (4) Are there reasons to believe that there are differences in values or belief that give rise to disagreement? (5) Is the patient's decisional capacity subtly impaired by psychiatric problems (such as depression or psychosis) or by medical problems (such as encephalopathy)?

RECOMMENDATION. In this case, we accept as ethically permissible the unauthorized treatment of a patient who appears to have mental capacity. We do so on the basis of the sliding scale explained earlier. The clinician's strong suspicion that the patient's medical condition has rendered him temporarily incapacitated to make a reasonable decision in his own best interest and the urgent need for life-saving and health-preserving intervention, support the decision to intervene.

Subsequent inquiry revealed that Mr. Cure's brother had nearly died 10 years earlier from an anaphylactic reaction to penicillin. But while in the emergency department, Mr. Cure did not, and could not, recall this event and probing did not uncover it. Mention of antibiotics had triggered a psychological response of fear and denial, which manifested itself in a refusal without reason. The circumstances of his particular illness drew the physicians in the direction of rapid treatment. Even though they made an effort to uncover the source of the problem, they failed to do so, and urgent need for treatment took priority.

This case illustrates that physicians are often pressured by circumstances to make decisions before all relevant information is known. The rightness or wrongness of the clinical decision always must be assessed with respect to the clinician's knowledge at the time of the decision. One can only strive to render decisions that are as fully informed and analyzed as the circumstances permit.

CASE III. Mrs. D., aged 77, is brought to the emergency department by a neighbor. Her left foot is gangrenous. She has lived alone for the last 12 years and is known by friends and by her doctor to be intelligent and independent. Her mental abilities are relatively intact, but she is becoming quite forgetful and is sometimes confused. On her last two visits to her doctor, she consistently called him by the name of her former physician, who is now dead. On being told that the best medical option for her problem is amputation of her foot, she adamantly refuses, although she insists she is aware of the consequences and accepts them. She calmly tells her doctor (whom she again calls by the wrong name) that she wants to be buried whole. He considers whether to seek judicial authority to treat her.

COMMENT. Mrs. D.'s mild dementia casts doubt on her ability to make an autonomous judgment. However, persons whose mental performance is somewhat abnormal should not automatically be disqualified as decision makers. Persons may not be well oriented to time and place and still understand the issue confronting them. The central test of a person's capacity is evidence that they understand the nature of an issue, and the consequences of any choice related to that issue. It is also possible to place any choice in the context of a person's own life history and values and ask whether the particular choice seems consistent with these. This is sometimes called the *authenticity* of the choice. Although ethicists argue over this as a criterion of mental capacity, it can often be a helpful clinical guide in evaluating the autonomy of the choice.

RECOMMENDATION. Mrs. D.'s clear assertions and the broader evidence of her life and values suggest that she has adequate decisional capacity to make an autonomous choice. Her physician does not need to seek a judicial determination of incompetence. Treatment of Mrs. D. should be limited to appropriate medical management, which, in this case, would be pain and symptom control and advance care planning.

CASE III. (Continued). Mrs. D. comes to the emergency department as described previously. In this version of the case, however, she adamantly denies that she has any medical problem. Although the toes of her left foot are necrotic and gangrenous tissue extends above the ankle, she insists that she is in perfect health and has been taking her daily walk every day, even this morning. Her neighbor asserts that Mrs. D. has been housebound for at least a week.

RECOMMENDATION. In this version, Mrs. D. shows definite signs of decisional incapacity. She denies her infirmity and her need for care, and appears to be delusional. She has given no previous directions about care. In Mrs. D.'s best interests, the appointment of a guardian should be sought who would then participate in considering and authorizing surgery. If Mrs. D's condition requires immediate surgical intervention, it should be considered an emergency (see Section 2.4.3).

2.2.5 Delirium, Confusion, and Waxing and Waning Capacity

Decisional capacity is often compromised by the pathological condition called *delirium*, that is, a disturbance of consciousness characterized by disorientation to place and persons, distraction, disorganized thinking, inattentiveness or hypervigilance, agitation or lethargy, and sometimes by perceptual disturbance, such as hallucinations. Delirium is usually of abrupt onset and variable in manifestation. It often accompanies trauma, sudden illness, and is not uncommon in the elderly. Also, in the so-called sundowner syndrome, a patient's mental capacity waxes and wanes: early in the day the person may appear clear and oriented but later be assessed as confused.

CASE. Mr. Care, with multiple sclerosis (MS), is now hospitalized. In the morning, he converses intelligibly with doctors, nurses, and family. In the afternoon, he confabulates and is disoriented to place and time. In both conditions, he expresses various preferences about care that are sometimes contradictory. In particular, when questioned in the morning about surgical placement of a tube to prevent aspiration, he refuses the placement; in the afternoon, however, he speaks confusedly and repeatedly about having the tube placed.

RECOMMENDATION. Unlike coma or dementia, delirium can be variable in presentation. Mr. Care's waxing and waning of mental status manifests the variability of delirium. In general, a delirious patient should be considered to have impaired capacity. If, however, the patient expresses consistent preferences during periods of clarity, it is not unreasonable to take them seriously. Still, supportive evidence about those preferences should be sought before they are taken as definitive.

2.2.6 Question Three—If Mentally Capable, What Preferences About Treatment Is the Patient Stating?

Most commonly, patients accept the recommendations of physicians. However, it is necessary to recall that it is patients who run the risks of the intervention. Even when an intervention promises a notable benefit, the patient may decide to decline the intervention. The prospective benefit may not fit into the patient's personal values and beliefs or its risks seem to great. In principle, when a patient with capacity to decide refuses recommended treatment, that refusal must be respected. In practice, the ethical problem may be complex. Thus, clinical situations arise when beliefs and values challenge the physician's recommendations.

2.2.7 Competent Refusal of Treatment by Persons with Capacity to Choose

Persons who are well informed and have decisional capacity sometimes refuse recommended treatment. If the recommended treatment is elective or if the consequences of refusal are minor, ethical problems are unlikely. However, if care is judged necessary to save life or to prevent serious consequences, physicians may be confronted with an ethical problem: does the physician's responsibility to help the patient ever override the patient's freedom to choose? The ethical principle of respect for autonomy, supported generally by American law, requires that refusal of care by a competent and informed adult should be respected, even if that refusal would lead to serious harm to the individual. The patient's refusal of well-founded recommendations is often difficult for the conscientious physician to accept. It is made more difficult when the patient's refusal, while competent, seems deliberately contrary to the patient's own welfare.

Lo B. Refusal of treatment by persons competent, informed patients. In: Lo B, ed. *Resolving Ethical Dilemmas. A Guide for Clinicians.* 4th ed. Philadelphia, PA: Lippincott Williams & Wilkins; 2009:83–87.

CASE I. Elizabeth Bouvia, a 28-year-old woman, was quadriplegic due to cerebral palsy. She also had severe arthritis. She is intelligent and articulate and, despite her disabilities, earned a college degree. While hospitalized for treatment of arthritic pain, the physicians determined that she was not getting sufficient nutrition by only taking food orally. A nasogastric tube was placed contrary to her wishes. She sought a court order to have the nasogastric tube removed. Although the trial court ruled in favor of the physicians and the hospital, the California Court of Appeals upheld her right to refuse tube feeding. The court said, "The right to refuse medical treatment is basic and fundamental. It is recognized as part of the right of privacy protected by both the state and federal constitutions. Its exercise requires no one's approval. It is not merely one vote subject to being overridden by medical opinion."

Bouvia v Superior Court (California Court of Appeals, 1986).

COMMENT. We cite *Bouvia v Superior Court* because it is a paradigm case of refusal of treatment by a competent person. Although a legal pronouncement, it conforms to the common interpretation of the ethical principle of autonomy.

CASE II. Ms. T.O. is a 64-year-old surgical nurse who had a resection for cancer of the right breast 5 years ago. She visited her physician again after discovering a 2-cm mass in the left breast. She agrees to a treatment program that includes lumpectomy, radiation therapy, and 6 months of chemotherapy. After her first course of chemotherapy, during which she experienced considerable toxicity, she informs her physician that she no longer wants any treatment. After extensive discussions with her physician and with her two daughters, she reaffirms her refusal of adjuvant therapy.

CASE III. Mr. S.P., the patient with aortic stenosis described in Section 2.1.7, Case II, has cardiac symptoms that indicate the need for coronary angiography. After hearing his physician explain the urgency for this procedure and its benefits and risks, he decides he does not want it.

COMMENT AND RECOMMENDATION. In Case I, Ms. T.O. makes a competent refusal of treatment. She is well informed and exhibits no evidence of any mental incapacitation. Even though the physician might consider the chances for prolonging disease-free survival better with chemotherapy, Ms. T.O. values her risks and chances differently. Her refusal should be respected. The physician should continue to observe Ms. T.O., particularly for the next several months during which a change of mind in favor of adjuvant therapy would still be beneficial. In Case II, Mr. S.P. is also competent. His refusal, even though it seems contrary to his interests, is an expression of his autonomy. It must be respected. That respect, however, also should encourage the physician to explore more fully the reasons for the refusal and to attempt to educate and persuade the patient. An early follow-up visit should be scheduled for both the patients to assure them that their physician remains supportive and concerned to help them deal with the consequences of their decision.

CASE IV. We have seen Mrs. Cope (see Section 2.2.4) admitted to the hospital for treatment of diabetic ketoacidosis with insulin, fluids, electrolytes, and antibiotics. That treatment was initiated over her objections but was authorized by her surrogate, Mr. Cope, who advised that her objections were the result of metabolic encephalopathy. After 24 hours, she awakens, talks appropriately with her family, and recognizes and greets her physician. She does not remember having been brought to the emergency department.

She now complains to the nurse and physician about pain in her right foot. Examination of the foot reveals that it is cold and mottled in color, and no pulses can be felt in the right leg distal to the right femoral artery. Doppler studies confirm arterial insufficiency. A vascular surgery consultation recommends an emergency arteriogram to examine the leg arteries. The benefits and risks of the procedure are explained, as well as the risks, including impairment of renal function. Mrs. Cope declines arteriography. The surgeons explain to her that they cannot do angioplasty and stenting unless they know what vessels are involved. The surgeons warn the patient that she faces a greater risk of losing her leg than a risk of losing renal function. Mrs. Cope participates in these discussions, asking appropriate questions, and acknowledging the doctors' comments. She again declines to have the arteriography.

COMMENT. Although 24 hours ago, Mrs. Cope was clearly decisionally incapacitated and was properly treated for pneumonia and ketoacidosis, despite her insistence to be left alone, the current situation is entirely different. She has now regained decisional capacity, can understand the situation, can consider the risks and benefits, and make up her mind. Her physician, nurses, and the consulting vascular surgeon agree that her decision is unwise—the low risk of worsening renal function is more than compensated for by the substantial benefit of saving her leg. Mrs. Cope does not agree. Her family is divided, some siding with the doctors and some with Mrs. Cope.

RECOMMENDATION. Mrs. Cope's decision must be respected. Efforts can be made to persuade her otherwise; time can be given for reconsideration. Still, Mrs. Cope shows no signs of incapacity and has the legal and moral right to make the decision that seems to her suitable. That decision may not be the best one from the viewpoint of medical indications, but law and ethics require respect for the patient's preferences in such circumstances.

2.2.8 Refusals Due to Religious Beliefs and Cultural Diversity

Certain religious groups hold beliefs about health, sickness, and medical care. Sometimes such beliefs will influence the patient's preferences about care in ways that providers might consider imprudent or dangerous. Similarly, persons from cultural traditions differing from the prevailing culture may view the medical practices of the prevailing culture as strange and even repugnant. In both cases, providers will be faced with the problem of reconciling a clinical judgment that seems reasonable to them and even an ethical judgment that seems obligatory, with a patient's preference for a different course of action. We offer here some general comments about this issue.

(a) Some clinicians who encounter unfamiliar beliefs may consider these beliefs "crazy" and even assume that anyone who holds them must suffer from impaired capacity. This response is wholly unjustified: it reveals bias and ignorance. The mere fact of adherence to an unusual belief is not, in and of itself, evidence of incapacity. In the absence of clinical signs of incapacity, such persons should be considered capable of choice.

(b) In institutions with a high volume of patients from a particular religious or cultural tradition should foster "cultural capacity." They should provide opportunities for providers to educate themselves about cultural beliefs. Cultural mediators, such as clergy or educated persons who can explain the beliefs and communicate with those who hold them, should be available. Competent translators should also be available for language problems. It should be noted, however, that the fact that a person speaks the same language or comes from the same country or religion as the patient does not guarantee competence as a translator or intermediary. Also, cultural stereotypes should be avoided; there are individuals from particular cultures who depart, in their values, preferences, and lifestyle, from the predominant mode of their cultures.

(c) To the extent possible, a treatment course that is acceptable to the patient and provider alike should be negotiated. It is first necessary to discover the common goals that are sought by the patient and the physician, and then to settle on mutually acceptable strategies to attain those goals. The appropriate ethical response to a genuine conflict is dependent on the circumstances of the case.

CASE I. A traditional Navajo man, 58 years old, is brought by his daughter to a community hospital. He is suffering severe angina. Studies show that he is a candidate for cardiac bypass surgery. The surgeon discusses the risks of surgery and says that there is a slight risk the patient may not wake up from surgery. The patient listens silently, returns home, and refuses to return to the hospital. His daughter, who is a trained nurse, explains, "The surgeon's words were very routine for him, but, for my dad, it was like a death sentence."

Carrese JA, Rhodes LA. Western bioethics on the Navajo Reservation. *JAMA.* 1995;274:826–829.

Singer PA, Viens AM. Section IX: Religious and cultural perspectives in bioethics. In: Singer PA, Viens AM, eds. *Cambridge Textbook of Bioethics*. New York, NY: Cambridge University Press; 2008:379–444.

COMMENT. This case represents a conflict between the duty of truthful disclosure and respect for the culturally diverse beliefs of the patient. In Navajo culture, language has the power to shape reality. Therefore, the explanation of possible risks is a prediction that the undesirable events are likely to occur. In Navajo culture, persons are accustomed to speak always in positive ways and to avoid speaking about evil or harmful things. The usual practice of informed consent, which requires the disclosure of risks and adverse effects, can cause distress and drive patients away from needed care. Similar reservations about the frankness of informed consent are found in other cultures. This issue will be discussed again in Topic Four, where we cover the role of the family (see Section 4.2.2).

RECOMMENDATION. Physicians who understand this feature of Navajo life would shape their discussions in accordance with the expectations of the patient. The omission of negative information, even though it would be unethical in dealing with a non-Navajo patient, is appropriate. This ethical advice rests on the fundamental value that underlies the rule of informed consent, namely, respect for persons, which requires that persons be respected, not as abstract individuals, but as formed within the values of their cultures.

CASE II. Mr. G. comes to a physician for treatment of peptic ulcer. He says he is a Jehovah's Witness. He is a firm believer and knows his disease is one that may eventually require administration of blood. He shows the physician a signed card affirming his membership and denying permission for blood transfusion. He quotes the biblical passage on which he bases his belief:

I (Jehovah) said to the children of Israel, "No one among you shall eat blood, nor shall any stranger that dwells among you eat blood."

(Leviticus 17: 12)

The physician inquires of her Episcopal clergyman about the interpretation of this passage. He reports that no Christian denomination except the Jehovah's Witnesses takes this text to prohibit transfusion. The physician considers that her patient's preferences impose an inferior standard of care. She wonders whether she should accept this patient under her care.

COMMENT. As a general principle, the unusual beliefs and choices of other persons should be tolerated if they pose no threat to other parties. The patient's preferences should be respected, even though they appear mistaken to others. The following general considerations apply to this case:

(a) Jehovah's Witnesses cannot be considered incapacitated to make choices unless there is clinical evidence of such incapacity. On the contrary, these persons are usually quite clear about their belief and its consequences. It is a prominent part of their faith, insistently taught and discussed. While others may consider it irrational, adherence to it is not, in itself, a sign of incompetence.

(b) Courts have almost unanimously upheld the legal right of adult Jehovah's Witnesses to refuse life-saving transfusions. If, however, unusual beliefs pose a threat to others, it is ethically permissible and may be obligatory to prevent harm by means commensurate with the imminence of the threat and the seriousness of the harm. Courts have consistently intervened to order blood transfusions for the minor children of Jehovah's Witnesses. Courts were once inclined to order transfusion for a parent whose death would leave children orphaned but now rarely do so because alternative care for children is usually available.

(c) The refusal of transfusion includes whole blood, packed red blood cells, white blood cells, plasma, and platelets. This faith forbids autotransfusion. It may allow administration of blood fractions, such as immune globulin, clotting factors, albumin, and erythropoietin. Dialysis and circulatory bypass techniques are permitted if they do not use blood products from others. It is advisable for the physician to determine exactly the content of a particular patient's belief from the patient, particularly before a situation arises in which blood or blood products may be a recommended treatment. Accurate knowledge of the teaching should be obtained from church elders.

Muramoto D. Jehovah's witness bioethics. In: Singer PA, Viens AM, eds. *The Cambridge Textbook of Bioethics.* New York, NY: Cambridge University Press; 2008:416–423.

(d) The refusal of blood transfusion by Jehovah's Witnesses differs in a significant way from refusal of all medical treatments. Jehovah's Witnesses acknowledge the reality of their illness and their desire to be cured or cared for; they simply reject one modality of care.

(e) Refusal of transfusion may lead the physician to consider whether transfusion is necessary in this clinical situation. A more careful consideration of the indications for transfusion has led to more conservative use of transfusion without serious harm. Some competent surgeons have undertaken to provide surgical procedures, including coronary artery bypass, for Jehovah's Witnesses without the use of blood transfusion; bloodless surgery centers have been instituted in some places.

(f) The physician's inquiry about the interpretation of the biblical passage is interesting. Presumably, she would feel more comfortable with a belief she knew was endorsed by her own religious tradition. The validity or truth of a religious belief is not relevant to the clinical decision. Instead, the sincerity of those who hold it and their ability to understand its consequences for their lives are the relevant issues in this type of case.

RECOMMENDATION. Mr. G.'s refusal should be respected for the following reasons:

(a) If a Jehovah's Witness comes as a medical patient, as did Mr. G., the eventual possibility of the use of blood should be discussed and a clear agreement should be negotiated between physician and patient about an acceptable manner of treatment. Under no circumstances should the physician resort to deception. A physician who, in conscience, cannot accept being held to an inferior or dangerous standard of care should not enter into a patient–physician relationship; or, if one already exists, should terminate it in the proper manner (see Section 2.5.6).

(b) If a Jehovah's Witness, who is known to be a confirmed believer, is in need of emergency care and refuses blood transfusion, the refusal ordinarily should be considered decisive. If a patient with diminished decisional capacity is known to clinicians as a Jehovah's Witness who has previously expressed his intention to refuse blood transfusion, clinicians may omit transfusion on grounds of an implied refusal. Witnesses often carry wallet cards stating their preference. If little is known about the patient and his or her status as a believer cannot be authenticated, treatment should be provided. In the face of uncertainty about personal preferences, it is our position that response to the patient's medical need should take ethical priority.

2.3 DECISION MAKING FOR THE MENTALLY INCAPACITATED PATIENT

Persons in need of medical care occasionally cannot make decisions on their own behalf. They can neither give consent to treatment nor refuse it. Their incapacity may have many causes. They may be unconscious or uncommunicative or both. They may be suffering from mental disabilities, either transitory, such as confusion or obtundation, or a chronic condition, such as dementia or a mental disease, for example, a psychotic depression that renders them mute. In such cases, alternative ways of decision making that do not rely on the direct participation of the patient, must be found. The first step in this alternative process is to inquire whether the patient has communicated any specific wishes about treatment prior to becoming mentally incapacitated. This question refers to Advance Planning and Advance Directives. The second step is to ask who should serve as the surrogate decision maker for the incapacitated patient.

Buchanan AE, Brock DW. *Deciding for Others: The Ethics of Surrogate Decision Making.* New York, NY: Cambridge University Press; 1989.

Lo B. Surrogate decision-making. In: Lo B, ed. *Resolving Ethical Dilemmas. A Guide for Physicians.* 4th ed. Philadelphia, PA: Lippincott Williams & Wilkins; 2009:101–106.

Pearlman R. Substitute decision making. In: Singer PA, Viens AM, eds. *The Cambridge Textbook of Bioethics.* New York, NY: Cambridge University Press; 2008:58–64.

2.3.1 Question Four—If Incapacitated, Has the Patient Expressed Prior Preferences?

The principle of autonomy requires that persons have the responsibility and the right to make decisions about how they should be treated during serious illness. Persons who are in good health rarely contemplate how serious disease or disability might affect them. However, serious illness often deprives the patient of the abilities to make decisions on their own behalf. In recent years, the concept of advance planning has been widely promoted as one solution to that problem.

2.3.2 Advance Planning

Advance planning encourages individuals to inform their physicians about the persons they most trust to decide on their behalf and how they would wish to be treated at a future time when they might be unable to participate in decisions about their care. The most important features of advance planning are discussion with one's family and a conference with one's doctor. The physician should document this conversation in the patient's record where it will be available in time of crisis.

In addition to these conversations, the wishes of the patient should be stated in legally acceptable documents, generally called "advance directives." There are several forms of advance directives: (1) the "durable (or medical) power of attorney for health care"; (2) the legal instrument entitled "Directive to Physicians" in statutes enacted by various states; and (3) the less formal "living will." Each of these forms is explained in the following paragraphs. Another form, called POLST (Physician Orders for Life-Sustaining Treatment), has been described in Section 1.3.6.

The idea of advance directives has become both familiar and accepted in ethics and in law. Medicare regulations require hospitals to provide patients with information about their rights under state law to accept or refuse recommended care and to formulate advance directives. In 1990, Congress passed the Patient Self-Determination Act requiring that all hospitals and other health care facilities receiving federal funds, such as Medicare and Medicaid payments, must ask patients at the time of admission whether they have advance directives. If they do, patients are asked to submit copies for their records; if they do not, they are to be informed that they have the right to prepare such a document. If the patient wishes to do so, most hospitals will provide a copy of a standard document and a packet of information. Physicians should encourage their patients to prepare advance directives; they should become familiar with the provisions of advance directives that are legally valid in their locale.

Although the legality of advance planning has been formalized by legislation and upheld by courts, physicians may still neglect to incorporate these methods of planning into their dealings with patients. Medical practice has been slow to respond to the preferences of terminally ill patients for less aggressive end-of-life care. Several empirical studies document that physicians are reluctant to discuss end-of-life issues with patients. In one large study (SUPPORT), systematic attempts to improve communication, information, and conversation between patients and physicians met with little success. Nor did the use of outcome data or patient preferences influence physician practices. End-of-life care, at least in the intensive care setting, is currently driven more by traditional hospital and physician practices to prolong life than by patient preferences, which are often difficult to discern when the patient is critically ill.

Davis J. Precedent autonomy: advanced directives and end of life care. In: Steinbock B, ed. *The Oxford Handbook of Bioethics.* New York, NY: Oxford University Press; 2009:349–374.

Lo B. Standards for decisions when patients lack decision-making capacity. In: Lo B, ed. *Resolving Ethical Dilemmas: A Guide for Clinicians.* 4th ed. Philadelphia, PA: Lippincott Williams & Wilkins; 2009:88–100.

SUPPORT Principal Investigators. A controlled trial to improve care for seriously ill hospitalized patients. *JAMA.* 1995;274:1591–1598.

The SUPPORT Project. Lessons for action. *Hastings Center Report.* 1995;25(6): S21–S22.

Tulsky JA, Emanuel LL, Martin DK, Singer PA. Advance care planning. In: Singer PA, Viens AM, eds. *The Cambridge Textbook of Bioethics.* New York, NY: Cambridge University Press; 2008:65–72.

2.3.3 The Durable Power of Attorney for Health Care

The most important element of advance planning is the authorization by the patient of a person who will make decisions on his or her behalf in case of mental incapacity. Such a person is commonly called a "designated decision-maker." There are several ways in which the designation of a decision maker can be given legal force.

State legislatures may pass a statute authorizing what is called "a durable power of attorney for health care." These statutes authorize individuals to appoint another person to act as their agent to make all health care decisions after they have become incapacitated. This person may be a relative or a friend. Most statutes require that this appointment be made in writing, although at least some states permit oral designation to be documented in the medical record of a surrogate decision-maker. These statutes give legal priority to the designated agent over all other parties, including next of kin. This clarifies the confusion that often exists about who in the family is the appropriate decision maker for an incapacitated relative. It also avoids the bureaucratic burdens and costs of a legal proceeding to appoint a guardian or conservator. A more complete discussion of the duties of these designated decision-makers appears in Section 2.4.

2.3.4 Documentation of Advance Planning: Advance Directives

The appointment of a designated decision-maker may be accompanied by a document that states, in more or less explicit terms, the forms of treatment that the patient wishes to have in the event of serious illness. Such a document is called an Advance Directive or a Directive to Physicians. Several different types of advance directives are presently in use. Although different in form and legal implications, all may be taken as evidence of a patient's preferences. These various types are:

(a) *Directive to Physicians in State Legislation.* These are statutes passed by state legislatures. These statutes affirm a person's right to make decisions regarding terminal care and provide directions about how that right can be effected after the loss of decision-making capacity. Typically, they contain a model (or sometimes mandatory) document called Directive to Physicians. These directives, which a patient can sign and give to the physician, are typically worded in this fashion: "If at any time I should have an incurable injury, disease, or illness certified to be a terminal condition by two physicians, and where the application of life-sustaining procedures would serve only to artificially prolong the moment of my death, and where my physician determines that my death is imminent whether or not life-sustaining procedures are used, I direct that such procedures be withheld or withdrawn, and that I be permitted to die naturally." Most such documents also contain a provision for the appointment of a designated decision-maker. Clinicians should know the specific features of the natural death acts of their states.

(b) *Living Wills.* Advance directives may be communicated by a person to physicians, family, and friends in less formal, less legalistic fashion than the statutory document described above. These less formal documents are generally called "living wills," (although this term is often applied to all advance care documents, including the statutory ones). One widely used document in earlier years contains the following words:

> If I become unable, by reason of physical or mental incapacity, to make decisions about my medical care, let this document provide the guidance and authority needed to make any and all such decisions. If I am permanently unconscious or there is no reasonable expectation of my recovery from a seriously incapacitating or lethal illness or condition, I do not wish to be kept alive by artificial means.

Some religious groups suggest particular forms of Living Wills for their adherents. Roman Catholics and Conservative Jews, for example, have forms that reflect their own doctrines on forgoing life support. Christian Science offers its members a document that supports their reluctance to accept medical interventions. Other forms of advance directives contain rather specific lists of particular procedures or conditions that the patient may wish to avoid or desire to have. A form called *Five Wishes* provides a document that allows persons to state their wishes about who will be the one to make decisions for them, the kind of medical treatment they want, how comfortable they want to be, how they want people to treat them, and what they wish their loved ones to know.

Aging with Dignity. Five Wishes. http://*www.agingwithdignity.org/five-wishes. php.*

Catholic Declaration on Life and Death. *http://www.flacathconf.org/* access date Jan 22, 2010.

Christian Science Advance Directive Addendum A. *www.canterburycrest.org/ downloads.html.*

Emanuel LL, Emanuel EJ. The medical directive: a new comprehensive advance care document. *JAMA.* 1989;261:3288–3292.

Hill TP, Shirley D. Choice in Dying. *A Good Death: Taking More Control at the End of Your Life.* Reading, MA: Addison-Wesley; 1992.

Jewish Medical Directives for Health Care, United Synagogue of Conservative Judaism. *http://www.uscj.org/Jewish_Advance_Medic6700html.*

(c) Finally, advance directives may be expressed in a personal note or letter that does not follow the forms described above. Such informal documentation allows a person to express in a more personal, and sometimes in a more precise way, their wishes. However, they may also be written very vaguely and, because of their unique nature, confuse those who must interpret them. Such documents, however, do have legal standing as evidence of a person's wishes in some jurisdictions. Even if there is no explicit legal recognition of personal documents, physicians should take account of them as expressions of their patient's preferences.

(d) Advance directive documents should be placed in a patient's hospital chart. Physicians caring for the patient should, if possible, discuss it with the patient or surrogate.

CASE I. Mr. Care, with MS, is now hospitalized because of aspiration pneumonia. He is alternatively obtunded and severely confused. He had given his physician a copy of the Directive to Physicians 4 years earlier. Now, in reviewing the directive, the physician notices the words (common in these documents), "the patient's death must be imminent, that is, death should be expected whether or not treatment is provided." Should the physician consider that if intubation is medically indicated, it should be withheld in accord with the patient's prior preferences?

CASE II. Mrs. A.T., a 70-year-old woman, very active and in good health, suffers a stroke after finishing a game of golf. She is admitted to the hospital unconscious and in respiratory distress. Studies show a brainstem and cerebellar infarct with significant edema involving the brainstem. She is provided ventilatory support. Her sister brings to the hospital a recently signed and witnessed Living Will. It contains the words, "I fear death less than the indignity of dependence and deterioration." The patient is currently unable to communicate. She is intubated and has cardiac arrhythmias. The neurologist believes that this patient has a reasonably good chance of recovery with uncertain functional deficit which could include gait disturbance. When he mentions to Mrs. A.T.'s sister that A.T. might have some gait disturbance, the sister responds, "I know A. wouldn't want to live like that." Should her physician, on becoming aware of the living will, extubate her? Should no-code orders be written?

CASE III. Mr W.W., a brilliant academic, appointed his wife as his designated agent for medical decisions and instructed her to decline artificial nutrition or hydration if he became severely demented. Mr. W.W. is now demented but maintains a pleasant affect, though he cannot converse and no longer recognizes family. He is now unable to feed himself or take food by mouth. The nursing home proposes to place a percutaneous endoscopic gastrostomy (PEG) tube to provide nutrition and hydration. His wife refuses to allow this; the nursing home administrator argues that Mr. W.W. is no longer the person who executed the advance directive but a "pleasantly demented individual" who may be enjoying his life.

RECOMMENDATION. In Case I, the physician may withhold intubation on the basis of the patient's advance directive. The words "whether or not treatment is provided" are a clumsy attempt to define the imminence of death. In this case, those words should not obstruct the fulfillment of Mr. Care's preferences, which seem quite clear. In Case II, withdrawing ventilatory support is premature given the facts of the case. It is as yet unclear whether Mrs. A.T. will suffer "the indignity of dependence and deterioration." However, if the patient's condition deteriorates, it may be appropriate to reconsider this option. If she recovers her ability to communicate and is competent, the exact meaning of her Living Will should be explored with her. In Case III, we believe Mr. W.W.'s instructions, and his wife's determination to follow his prior wishes should be respected even in his present state, because when he had the capacity, he obviously considered scenarios just such as his present situation. We believe that choices made on the basis of stable values should be honored.

COMMENT. Written advance directives are an important innovation in the expression of patient preferences. They allow persons to project their preferences into the future for consideration by those responsible for their care when they themselves are no longer capable of expressing preferences. However, advance directives may present some problems to those who must interpret them. They necessarily employ general expressions, such as "if there is no reasonable expectation of recovery" or the direction to forgo "artificial means and heroic measures." Such language requires interpretation in the setting of the case. Further, persons may have prepared these documents without much discussion or reflection, as they go through estate planning. In addition, they usually do not specifically indicate which of the various means of life-sustaining treatments the patient desires to forgo. Finally, some commentators raise the question, whether preferences expressed while a person enjoys decisional capacity should be honored after the patient has permanently lost such capacity. Although these documents are helpful as evidence about the patient's prior preferences and should be taken seriously, they do not replace timely discussion with patients and surrogates, as well as thoughtful and responsible interpretation in the particular case. Ethics consultation may also be helpful in interpreting advance directives.

2.4 SURROGATE DECISION-MAKERS

Crucial clinical decisions must often be made when a patient is very sick and unable to communicate his or her desires about care. Other persons speak on their behalf. Such persons are called *surrogates*. Traditionally, next of kin have been considered the natural surrogates, and clinicians have turned to family members for their permission to treat the patient. This practice has been tacitly accepted in Anglo-American law, but was rarely expressed in statutes.

2.4.1 Question Five—Who Is the Appropriate Surrogate to Make Decisions for the Incapacitated Patient?

In recent years, efforts have been made to clarify the determination of surrogates for medical decision making. Statutes authorize persons to appoint their own surrogates, or holders of durable powers of attorney (see Section 2.3.3). These appointed surrogates supercede any other party, including immediate family members. In addition, many states have enacted legislation that gives specific authority to certain family members, ranking them in priority (for example, first spouse, then parents, then children, then siblings, etc). These statutes avoid the need to seek judicial recourse, except in cases of conflict or doubt about legitimate decision-makers. Statutes of this sort are helpful in avoiding conflicting claims to authority. On the other hand, they may automatically appoint some party who is inappropriate. Finally, all states have provisions for the judicial appointment of guardians or conservators for those declared incompetent by a judge.

2.4.2 The Standards for Surrogate Decisions

The decisions of surrogates are guided by definite standards. There are two sorts of standard. The first is called "substituted judgment": when the patient's preferences are known, the surrogate must use knowledge of these preferences in making medical decisions. The second is called "the best interest standard": when the patient's preferences are not known, the surrogate's judgment must promote the best interests of the patient.

(a) *Substituted Judgment. "Substituted judgment" is when a surrogate relies on known preferences of the patient to reach a conclusion about medical treatment.* This is used in two situations: (1) where the patient has previously expressed her preferences explicitly, and (2) where the surrogate can reasonably infer the patient's preferences from past statements or actions.

The first situation is the most straightforward and occurs when the patient has previously expressed preferences concerning the course of action she would desire in the present circumstances. Whether the patient recorded these preferences in writing or merely informed another person of the preferences orally, the surrogate should follow the patient's preferences as closely as possible. In effect, the surrogate is not making medical decisions for the patient, but is merely giving effect to decisions the patient would have made for herself. Courts typically apply this standard in situations where the patient's preferences are known. In a landmark legal case, *In the Matter of Karen Quinlan* (1976), the New Jersey Supreme Court was faced with the difficult decision of whether to permit the withdrawal of a respirator from a young woman in a persistent vegetative state with no chance for recovery. Before the incident that led to her impaired condition, the patient had made statements indicating that she would not want to be kept alive by extraordinary means if there was little chance for recovery. The court relied on these statements in applying the substituted judgment standard to permit her legal guardian to order the removal of the respirator.

When the patient has not specifically stated what she would want, a surrogate should base his decision on familiarity with the patient's values and beliefs. Obviously, only individuals with a close association to the patient are suitable as surrogates when this sort of judgment is called for. Surrogates must be careful to avoid the common pitfall of injecting their own values and beliefs into the decision-making process. Only the patient's values and beliefs are relevant to the substituted judgment decision.

Two important legal cases illustrate the importance of surrogate decision-makers and substituted judgment. In the case of Nancy Cruzan (1990), the United States Supreme Court was confronted with a request by her father, who was her legal guardian to remove artificial nutrition and hydration tubes from a young woman in a chronic vegetative state. The patient had previously made statements to her roommate that she would not want to continue her life if she could not live "halfway normally." The Court, while endorsing the substituted judgment standard, declined to order the removal of the tubes, because the evidence about the patient's preferences failed to meet Missouri's evidentiary standards. The Court ruled that each state can adopt its own evidentiary standards in such cases. When the case was sent back to the trial court, the judge ruled that her roommate's testimony along with additional testimony from her friends constituted clear and convincing evidence of Nancy's preferences. Artificial nutrition and hydration were terminated at the request of her father and she died in 2 weeks.

In the widely publicized case of Terri Schiavo (2005), Ms. Schiavo had been in a chronic vegetative state for 15 years, fed by a feeding tube. Her husband, who had been judicially appointed as her legal guardian, was authorized to make a substituted judgment on her behalf. Mr. Schiavo asserted that his wife had expressed her preference not "to be kept alive on a machine." Her brother-in-law and sister-in-law corroborated this testimony, which was accepted as clear and convincing evidence by all of the courts that adjudicated the case. Life support was discontinued despite numerous objections raised by her parents, her siblings, and many political figures. These two cases are described more fully in Section 3.3.7.

It must be acknowledged that many studies have shown that surrogates often mistakenly believe that they know what their family member would have wanted. One study, for example, showed that surrogates predicted the patient's preferences with 68% accuracy. Even then, the surrogates were more accurate than physicians. A substituted judgment standard, then, cannot always be taken at face value. The surrogates' information should be discussed, probed, and checked against other sources of information. At best, information derived from surrogates can help to formulate a picture of the values and beliefs of the patient. Still, legitimate surrogates must be permitted to make these decisions as long as clinicians believe they are acting in good faith.

(b) *Best Interests. If the patient's own preferences are unknown or are unclear, the surrogate must consider the best interests of the patient. This requires that the surrogate's decision must promote the individual's welfare, which is defined as making those choices, namely, about relief of suffering, preservation or restoration of function, and the extent and sustained quality of life, that reasonable persons in similar circumstances would be likely to choose.* The concept of best interest is discussed in connection with quality of life, in Section 3.0.7.

Beauchamp TL, Childress JF. A framework of standards for surrogate decision making. In: Beauchamp TL, Childress JF, eds. *Principles of Biomedical Ethics*. 6th ed. New York, NY: Oxford University Press; 2009: 135–140.

Shalowitz DI, Garrett-Hayes E, Wendler D. The accuracy of surrogate decision makers. *Arch Intern Med.* 2006;166:493–497.

2.4.3 Implied Consent

In life-threatening emergencies, patients may be unable to express their preferences or give their consent because they are unconscious or in shock. No surrogate may be available. In such situations, it has become customary for physicians to presume that the patient would give consent if able to do so, because the alternative would be death or severe disability. This is sometimes called *implied consent*. The patient is not, of course, giving consent; the physician is presuming that the patient would consent, if they could. From the ethical point of view, the principle of beneficence, which prescribes that a person has a duty to assist someone in serious need of help, is the ethical justification for emergency treatment of the incapacitated person. It is a reasonable presumption that a person would, if they could, accept help in a critical situation. Implied consent also provides the physician with a legal defense against a subsequent charge of battery, although it may not defend against charges of negligence if the emergency treatment falls below acceptable standards of care; for example, a physician incorrectly performs a Heimlich maneuver, thereby breaking ribs and puncturing a lung.

2.4.4 Decisions for Patients Who Lack Surrogates

A patient who has lost decisional capacity may have no person who can be identified as a surrogate. The term "unbefriended or unrepresented patient" is sometimes used.

CASE. An elderly woman collapses in a bus station. She is carrying no identity. She is taken to the emergency department. She is badly malnourished with end-stage liver disease. She also has pneumonia. She is intubated, on grounds of an emergency implied consent. She remains stuporous. After 3 days in the ICU, she develops hepatorenal syndrome and renal failure. Emergency dialysis is initiated on grounds of implied consent. However, after a week, question arises about terminating respiratory support and dialysis, since her underlying disease is liver failure and, due to age and comorbidities, she is not a candidate for transplantation.

COMMENT. A legal proceeding to appoint a guardian for this patient can be instigated. The Hospital Social Work Department is adept at this task. However, often it takes considerable time and, as in this case, the critical need for a surrogate emerged slowly. There is no agreed approach to a problem of this sort. If legal recourse is not feasible, ethics committees may review the case and, on the basis of principles of beneficence and nonmaleficence, advise clinicians regarding treatment. However, ethics committees are hospital entities, and as such, open to allegations of conflict of interest. It is important that hospitals formulate a policy that would provide for a decision-making process in which conflict is reduced, for example, by having an outside consultant or by submitting the case to another ethics committee.

2.4.5 Statutory Authority to Treat

In all jurisdictions, statutes exist that authorize psychiatrists to restrain mentally ill persons who are dangerous to themselves or others for psychiatric treatment against their will. These statutes pertain to persons who are suffering from mental disease, and the treatment authorized is treatment *only* for mental disease. In some situations, both mental disease and medical problems may be present. These situations of dual diagnoses deserve special consideration.

CASE. A 75-year-old veteran of the Vietnam War is brought to the hospital by a friend. He has a long history of mental disease and alcohol addiction. He has been drinking and is hallucinating that Viet Cong are attacking him.

He is breathless, has fainted twice in the last hour, and is incontinent of urine. He says his heart is breaking through his chest. Still, he says he must leave the hospital because it is being bombed. The admitting resident writes in the chart, "I noted hallucinations and psychotic ideation; I am putting the patient on a medical hold and keeping him in the hospital for observation. Diagnosis: paroxysmal supraventricular tachycardia. Medications: haloperidol, digitalis. Further evaluation: assess electrolytes."

COMMENT. The question is whether the statutory authorization for involuntary hospitalization allows medical treatment as well as treatment for mental illness. The answer is, it does not. The statutes refer to the treatment of mental illness alone as the justification for involuntary commitment. If medical treatment is needed, the patient must consent or, if unable to do so, a legally authorized decision-maker must be appointed. If medical treatment is needed for a life-saving emergency, implied consent suffices.

RECOMMENDATION. The emergency department resident should immediately request psychiatric consultation. The consulting psychiatrist will examine the patient and, having made a diagnosis of paranoid schizophrenia, may authorize involuntary commitment for treatment of this mental disorder. The emergency department resident does not have this authority. The term *medical hold* is sometimes used to describe this procedure but it is misleading for two reasons: physicians, other than psychiatrists, cannot "hold" patients, and only psychiatric treatments may be administered.

2.5 FAILURE TO COOPERATE IN THE THERAPEUTIC RELATIONSHIP

A therapeutic relationship is constituted by two parties cooperating in the effort to achieve the goals of medicine, that is, curing and caring. Both parties can withdraw, partially or totally, willingly or unwillingly, from this cooperative effort. Patients may give consent to a treatment recommendation but fail to follow the recommended treatment. At the same time, they express a desire to continue the therapeutic relationship. This situation was once commonly called "noncompliance," although that term is seldom used today because of its paternalistic overtones. The problem, whatever it is called, can create persistent ethical dilemmas for all involved. Also, there are occasions on which physicians and other health professionals are unwilling to provide some forms of care. This raises the ethical problem of conscientious objection.

2.5.1 Question Six—Is the Patient Unwilling or Unable to Cooperate with Medical Treatment? If So, Why?

Physicians have the responsibility to recommend to patients a course of treatment or behavior that would, in the physician's best judgment, help the patient. Patients have the right to be informed of the benefits and risks associated with these recommendations and to accept them or refuse them. These rights and responsibilities are in principle quite clear. However, patients may fail to act on their physician's recommendations, yet continue to seek the care of the physician. In place of the terms "noncompliance" or "nonadherence," we use the expression "failure to cooperate with medical recommendations." The problem posed to physicians is how they should perform their ethical responsibilities to patients who ask for help but for some reason do not, or cannot, follow the course of treatment that is offered.

2.5.2 Failure to Cooperate with Medical Recommendations

A patient may not cooperate with recommended treatment for many reasons. The following cases represent two examples of this very complex problem.

CASE I. Ms. Cope is a 42-year-old woman with insulin-dependent diabetes who, despite good compliance with an insulin and dietary regimen, experienced frequent episodes of ketoacidosis and hypoglycemia that necessitated repeated hospitalizations and emergency room visits. For the past few years, her diabetes has been better controlled. She has been actively involved in her diabetic program, has been scrupulous about her eating habits, and has maintained ideal body weight. Twenty-one years after the onset of diabetes, she appears to have no functional impairment from her disease.

Three years ago, Ms. Cope went through a stormy divorce and lost an executive position. She has gained 60 lb and has become negligent about her insulin medication. She has also started to drink alcohol excessively. During these years, she has required frequent admissions to the hospital for diabetic complications, including (1) ketoacidosis, (2) traumatic and poorly healing foot ulcers, and (3) alcohol-related problems. While in the hospital, her diabetes is easier to manage but even in the hospital, she is frequently found in the cafeteria eating excessively. On two admissions, blood alcohol levels in excess of 200 mg/dL were detected. Soon after discharge from the hospital, her diabetic control lapses.

Her physician is frustrated. He blames the recurring medical problems on the patient's unwillingness to participate actively in her own care by losing weight, taking insulin regularly, and giving up alcohol. The patient promises to change her lifestyle, but on discharge from the hospital, she relapses almost immediately. The physician urges her to seek psychiatric consultation. She agrees. The psychiatrist suggests a behavior modification program, which proves unsuccessful.

After 10 years of working closely with this patient, the physician considers withdrawing from the therapeutic relationship, because he senses he is no longer able to help the patient. "Why keep this up?" he says to the patient. "It's useless. Whatever I do, you undo." The patient resists this suggestion. She complains that the physician is abandoning her. Does persistent failure to comply with medical advice justify an ethical decision to withdraw from a case?

COMMENT. The following comments are relevant to this question:

(a) Patients such as Ms. Cope are very frustrating to those who attempt to care for them. Occasionally, the physician will accuse the patient (in words or in attitude) of being irresponsible. The patient engages constantly and, apparently, willfully in behavior that poses a serious risk to health and even to life. Such patients place great strain on the doctor–patient relationship; often the accommodation between doctor and patient founders because of the strain.

(b) The accusation of irresponsibility can be an example of the ethical fallacy of "blaming the victim"; the actual fault may lie with a more powerful party who finds a way to place the blame for his own failure on the ones who suffer its effects. The apparent irresponsibility of patients may result from the failure of a physician to educate, support, and convey a personal concern and interest in the patient. Even more, persons may be rendered incapable of caring responsibly for themselves by the way their physician deals with them. An excessive paternalism may stifle responsibility. Although Ms. Cope's physician did not have these faults and had made solicitous efforts to support Ms. Cope, this problem may lie behind many cases of a patient's failure to cooperate.

RECOMMENDATIONS.

(a) It is important to determine whether and to what extent the patient is acting voluntarily or involuntarily. Much uncooperative behavior is voluntary. Patients either choose to ignore the regimen in favor of other behaviors they value more than health (a goal that, in an asymptomatic disease, may not seem very urgent or immediate), or fail to cooperate because of such factors as irregular routine, complicated regimen, habitual forgetfulness, or poor explanation by the physician. Some noncompliance is nonvoluntary, arising from profound emotional disturbance or psychological disabilities and ambivalence.

(b) If the physician judges that noncooperation is voluntary, a result of the patient's persistence in voluntary health risks, then reasonable efforts at rational persuasion should be undertaken. If these fail, it is ethically permissible for the physician to adjust therapeutic goals and do the best in the circumstances. It is also ethically permissible to withdraw from the case, after advising the patient how to obtain care from other sources. This should be done in accord with the ethical and legal standards noted in Section 2.5.6.

(c) If noncooperation is the result of a psychological disorder, the physician has a strong ethical obligation to remain with the patient, adjusting treatment plans to the undesirable situation. Professional assistance in treating the disorder should be sought. The physician may experience great frustration, but the frustration is not, in itself, sufficient to justify leaving the patient.

CASE II. Ms. Cope is admitted for inpatient treatment of obesity with a protein-sparing modified fasting regimen. She was found repeatedly in the cafeteria cheating on the diet. Clinicians made reasonable efforts to persuade her to change her behavior. A decision was made to discharge her. She protested vigorously.

RECOMMENDATION. It is ethically permissible for the physician to terminate therapeutic efforts and to discharge the patient from the hospital. The goals of therapy are unachievable because of the patient's failure to participate in the program. This decision may be the culmination of a long history of failure to cooperate leading to the physician's decision to withdraw from the care of Ms. Cope. Also, a return to prior lifestyle, while inadvisable and potentially harmful, is not the direct cause of harm to the patient.

Failure to cooperate in a medical regimen is a most complex problem that may be rooted in psychological, social, or economic features of the patient's life, as well as in the difficulties of understanding and navigating the medical system. It is incumbent on physicians to understand the deep roots of this problem.

2.5.3 The Disruptive Patient

On occasion, persons who are under care in a health care facility may cause serious disruption and even endanger other patients. At the same time, they may desire to continue in treatment. Physicians who encounter such challenging patients may be concerned that discharging them because of the danger posed to others or the disruptions caused may induce serious harm, even death, for the patient.

CASE. Mr. R.A., an intravenous drug addict, is admitted for the third time in 3 years with a diagnosis of infective endocarditis. Three years ago, he required mitral valve replacement for *Pseudomonas* endocarditis, and 1 year ago, he required replacement of the prosthetic valve after he developed *Staphylococcus aureus* endocarditis. He now is admitted again with *S. aureus* endocarditis of the prosthetic valve.

After 1 week of antibiotic therapy, he continues to have positive blood culture results. One cardiac surgeon refuses to operate, saying that the patient is a recidivist and that correcting his drug addiction is futile. Another surgeon agrees to operate on him. Mr. R.A. consents to open heart surgery to replace again the infected prosthetic mitral valve. Postoperatively, for 10 days he is cooperative with his management and antibiotic treatment. While on this treatment, he becomes afebrile and blood culture data are negative. Plans are in place for his discharge, with venous access for antibiotics.

He then begins to behave erratically. He leaves his room and stays away for hours, often missing his medications. On several occasions, a urine screening test demonstrates the presence of opiates and quinine, revealing that he is using illicit narcotics even while being treated for infective endocarditis. Two repeat blood culture tests now grow *S. aureus*. On two separate occasions, he verbally abuses two nurses who reprimand him for being away from his room. Several patients on the unit complain that he threatened them. Nurses suspect that he is also dealing drugs within the hospital. This information becomes known to the patient's physician; despite the fact that the patient's infective endocarditis has not been treated optimally, the physician asks him to leave the hospital immediately.

COMMENT. Considerations leading to an ethical justification of this decision are as follows:

(a) The patient's use of intravenous street drugs at the same time that his physicians were attempting to eradicate his infective endocarditis indicated that the likelihood of medical success in this case, both short-term and long-term, was not great. Physicians are not obliged to treat people who persist in actions that run counter to the goals of treatment.

(b) The patient wanted to be treated and, at the same time, continued his abusive behavior. The physicians are obliged to determine that the patient has the mental capacity to make such choices and that he was not suffering from a metabolic encephalopathy (see Section 2.2.3).

(c) Providers should try to understand the complex causes of his behavior and motivations. They should avoid "blaming the victim." Serious efforts should be made to counsel, to negotiate, and to develop "contracts" that make clear to him the consequences of his behavior. Early and repeated warnings should be issued. One identified provider should be responsible for dealing with this patient.

(d) In addition to his uncooperative behavior, which is harmful to himself, he disrupts the functioning of the hospital and impedes the care of other patients. This additional contextual feature provides an additional argument in favor of his discharge. The ethical basis of this argument is fairness: his behavior deprives other patients of rightful attention (see Section 4.5).

RECOMMENDATION. Clinicians should recognize that this patient's primary medical problem is not endocarditis, serious though that condition is. As the first surgeon noted, it is drug addiction. The focus of his treatment should shift to treatment for that problem. The management of addiction requires long-term outpatient care and support. Nevertheless, he is at risk of dying in the short term from another episode of infective endocarditis. In our opinion, he should be discharged with an indwelling venous line and with home nursing service to administer antibiotics. This is not optimal care, but it would provide reasonable care to this patient while protecting the interests of others. If he proves intractable, then it can be argued that efforts to manage his endocarditis by surgical means will not be effective and the patient may be discharged.

2.5.4 Signing Out Against Medical Advice

Mr. R.A. might simply walk out of the hospital, leaving even before physicians judge his treatment adequate. When patients choose to discharge themselves in this manner, most hospitals request them to sign a statement confirming that they are leaving against medical advice (AMA). The patients, however, cannot be forced to sign the statements; they have the right to leave at will. The document merely provides legal evidence that the patient's departure was voluntary, and that the patient was warned by the physician about the risks of leaving.

2.5.5 Conscientious Objection

The preferences of patients have significant moral authority and must be considered in every treatment decision. Even the preferences of decisionally incapacitated patients are relevant to the decisions of those who must act on their behalf. However, the authority of patients' preferences is not unlimited. The ethical obligations of physicians are defined not only by the wishes of their patients but also by the goals of medicine. Physicians have no obligation to perform actions beyond or contradictory to the goals of medicine, even when requested to do so by patients. Patients have no right to demand that physicians provide medical care that is contraindicated, such as unnecessary surgery or medically inappropriate drug regimens. Patients may not demand that physicians do anything illegal. For example, physicians must not provide certification of a disability that the patient does not have or fail to report at a patient's request a legally reportable communicable disease. Finally, physicians may refuse to accede to a patient's wishes when they believe that doing so will make them complicit in something they believe is immoral.

Traditionally, medical ethics has required physicians to abstain from moral judgments about their patients in regard to medical care. For example: (1) an emergency department physician is expected to provide competent care to both the wounded assailant of an elderly person and to the assaulted party; and (2) a physician should treat, without censure, venereal disease contracted in what the physician considers an immoral liaison. However, despite this professional neutrality, physicians and nurses have their own personal moral values. On occasion, they may be asked not merely to tolerate what they consider immorality but to participate in effecting what they consider an immoral action desired by the patient. For example: (1) a male patient requests a physician who considers transsexualism morally wrong to prescribe female estrogens to promote secondary female characteristics; and (2) a Catholic nurse is asked to participate in an abortion. This is described as *conscientious objection, which means a judgment formed on the basis of sincerely held moral values that participation in some particular action would be violating one's own moral standards.* A person should be able to articulate a reason for this judgment that refers to the underlying moral values. Traditionally, laws permitting abortion and laws permitting physician-assisted dying contain explicit exemptions for conscientious objection. However, providers may invoke conscientious objection in other situations that may be not only controversial but also not legally justified. For example, a pharmacist refuses to fill a valid prescription for a "morning after pill." A physician may conscientiously judge that a particular law is unethical. For example, a physician who is treating patients with AIDS is convinced that smoking marijuana relieves the pain and nausea of advanced illness, but state law prohibits prescription of medical marijuana.

Physicians and nurses may refuse to cooperate in actions they judge immoral on grounds of conscience. It is important, in forming one's conscience, to separate the moral values to which one is committed from personal distaste or prejudice. For example, a physician refuses to undertake the care of a Jehovah's Witness with a hemorrhagic diathesis on moral grounds, although, in fact, the physician does not want to take the risk that the patient may die from blood loss. Institutions and programs should establish policies about conscientious objection and make the policies as well as the state laws clear to those who work in that institution or program. The traditional ethics of conscientious objection require the objector to make clear his or her position in a public way and to accept the consequences of objection, such as legal liability for violation of a law.

2.5.6 Withdrawing from the Case and Abandonment of the Patient

At times, such as the case of Ms. Cope (see Section 2.5.2), the physician may serve the patient best by deciding to dissolve the physician–patient relationship. The physician's principal goal is to help patients in the care of their health. If this proves impossible, the physician may best demonstrate ethical responsibility by withdrawing from the case.

Physicians who terminate a relationship with a patient sometimes wonder whether they can be charged with abandonment. *Abandonment, in the legal sense, means that a physician, without giving timely notice, ceases to provide care for a patient who is still in need of medical attention or when the physician is dilatory and careless (e.g., failure to see the patient at a time of urgent need or failure to judge the patient's condition serious enough to warrant attention).* A charge of abandonment can usually be countered by showing that the patient did receive warning in sufficient time to arrange for medical care. The physician is not legally obliged to arrange for further care from another physician, although there is a legal obligation to provide full medical records to the new attending physician. If the physician does intend to maintain the relationship with the patient but will be unavailable for a time, there is a legal obligation to arrange for coverage by another physician. Failure to do so can be construed as abandonment.

A physician may withdraw from the care of a patient without legal risk. The decision to do so should meet ethical as well as legal standards. Physicians inherit an ethical tradition that requires them to undertake difficult tasks and even risks for the care of persons in need of medical attention. Inconvenience, provocation, or dislike are not sufficient reasons to exempt a physician from that duty. That obligation is, of course, limited by several conditions—if the patient absorbs excessive time and energy, drawing the physician away from other patients; if the patient is acting in ways to frustrate the attainable medical goals; or if the patient is endangering others by overt action—the ethical obligation to continue to care would be diminished. These conditions appear to be verified in the case of Mr. R.A. Finally, a physician may decline to provide nonbeneficial treatments or treatments contrary to conscience, as noted in Section 2.5.3.

2.5.7 Complementary/Alternative Medicine

Some persons seek health care from alternative providers outside or in addition to conventional scientific medicine. It is estimated that 1 out of 3 adult Americans make a total of 425 million visits to alternative providers—more than are made to primary care practitioners. These providers include naturopaths, homeopaths, chiropractors, acupuncturists, and practitioners of traditional Chinese, Indian, and Native American medicine. In several states, homeopathic and naturopathic doctors are licensed as medical practitioners. Methods include spiritual healing, physical manipulation, special diets, imaging, relaxation techniques, massage, and vitamin therapy, and attention is paid to nutrition, exercise, and stress reduction. These methods are described as *alternative* or *complementary* medicine (CAM). *Integrative medicine* designates programs that attempt to find and utilize the benefits of both alternative and orthodox medicine. Some prominent medical institutions have established programs in integrative medicine.

Adams KE, Cohen MH, Eisenberg D, Jonsen AR. Ethical considerations of complementary and alternative medical therapies in conventional medical settings. *Ann Intern Med.* 2002;137:660–664.
Cohen MH. Alternative and complementary medicine. In: Singer PA, Viens AM, eds. *The Cambridge Textbook of Bioethics.* New York, NY: Cambridge University Press; 2008:513–520.

CASE. A 64-year-old man has been under the care of a family physician for increasingly severe osteoarthritis. On one visit, he complains of dizzy spells. A workup reveals no specific cause for his dizziness. In discussing his arthritis, he tells his doctor that he gets some relief from mushroom tea. The physician has seen reports of illness caused by "kombucha tea," which, although called "mushroom tea," is actually a colony of bacteria and yeast fermented in sweetened tea. The physician questions the patient, and the patient reluctantly admits that he has been seeing a "natural healer" who sold him the concoction.

McNaughton C, Eidsness LM. Ethics of alternative therapies. *S D J Med.* 1995;48:209–211.

COMMENT. Many persons who visit alternative practitioners are also under the care of regular practitioners, using unconventional therapies as adjuncts rather than replacements of conventional therapy. Many of these patients do not inform their regular physician about their use of alternative treatment. Persons are often motivated to seek alternative treatments because they are less arduous and less costly than conventional treatments, or because patients are frustrated with the failure of conventional treatment to assuage problems such as chronic back pain, headache, insomnia, anxiety, and depression. Most conventional practitioners know little about alternative medicine, and many commonly disdain it and disparage its claims.

RECOMMENDATION.

(a) Conventional physicians should encourage their patients to reveal their use of alternative medications. They should refrain from disparaging remarks that can inhibit patients from speaking about what they fear will lead to anger or ridicule on the physician's part.

(b) Conventional physicians should try to attain a better understanding of the healing systems to which patients have recourse and to appreciate their beneficial features. Persons often take substances that are advertised or promoted on Web sites, without supervision of either alternative or regular physicians. This unsupervised medication regime may have adverse effects. For example, licorice, an herb used in many supplements promoted for relief of fatigue can lower serum potassium significantly; many supplements, such as fish oils, may affect coagulation. When regular practitioners see these effects, they may neither know that their patients are using these substances, nor understand their nature and risks. Patients should be asked whether they are using alternative medications. Consultation with an established CAM practitioner or program may be advisable. Reliable information about herbal medications can be found in the *Botanical Safety Handbook* (CRC Press) or at HerbMed www.herbmed.org.

(c) When patients are using alternative therapies for serious conditions to the neglect of demonstrated efficacious therapies or when they are using therapies that have toxic effects, physicians should carefully explain the consequences of such a course. A clumsy or uninformed approach may confirm patients in the use of inadvisable therapy rather than convert them to more appropriate ones.

(d) In serious conditions, where the use of alternative medicine may impede cure or be dangerous, the physician should ask the patient's permission to contact the alternative provider, explain the situation, and negotiate a program that will be acceptable to the patient as well as conformable to the ethics of the providers.

(e) Hospitals should develop policies that acknowledge the prevalence of alternative therapies and establish guidelines for acceptable collaboration between regular physicians and providers of alternative treatments.

2P PEDIATRIC NOTES

2.1P Authority of Parents and Consent of Minors

Children are considered incompetent under the law. The medical care of infants and children is authorized by the usual surrogates, namely, the parents of the child, or in unusual circumstances, by other parties authorized by law. In addition, the law designates the age at which young persons are deemed competent to consent. Two ethical issues about surrogacy for children may occur. First, it is sometimes necessary to determine the relevance and weight of parental preferences when these preferences conflict with the recommendations of providers. Second, children become capable of expressing their preferences at various ages. When they do express preferences, it is necessary to determine how reasonable and relevant these preferences are in matters of medical care. Finally, certain general exceptions to parental authority exist: special statutes give certain authority to minors to decide health care on their own.

Parental responsibility is a moral, social, and legal matter. It is commonly agreed that parents have the responsibility for the well-being of their children and that they have a wide range of discretion to determine the particular circumstances that this well-being will encompass. At the same time, parental discretion is not absolute. Infants and children are, in American law, considered persons, with certain interests and rights that must be acknowledged regardless of their parents' preferences. It is usually said that the best interests of the child set limits on the discretion of parents about the medical treatment of their offspring. Also, American society accepts, as an obligation, the protection of children from harm, even at the hands of their parents. Further, the welfare of children is taken as a serious social obligation.

As children become mature enough to articulate their preferences and reasons for them, they are entitled to increasing respect for these preferences. They are led toward responsible maturity by this respect and by education. However, it is sometimes difficult to decide how much respect to afford a child's preferences. It is difficult to discern how rational these preferences are because consequences, alternatives, and relative values are often not perceived clearly by children. Certain sorts of decisions made by nonadults have been codified in the law. Persons who are younger than the statutory age of consent (18 years in all states), may come to a physician on their own initiative. When their medical problem is not an emergency, such persons can be treated only with the consent of their parents or legal guardian, however, there are several exceptions to this rule.

(a) Almost all jurisdictions now have special provisions for the treatment of certain conditions without the consent of the minor's parents. These conditions usually include drug abuse and venereal disease (contraception, abortion, and mental illness are sometimes included, and at other times, specifically excluded). Most states permit minors to make decisions about contraception and abuse treatment, without parental permission.

(b) The emancipated minor is a young person who lives independently of parents, physically, financially, or otherwise. Married minors, those in the armed forces, or those living away at college are considered emancipated. They may request treatment and be treated without parental consent.

(c) "Mature minor" designates a person who is below statutory age and who is still dependent upon parents but who appears to make reasoned judgments. These young persons pose something of a quandary to the physician from whom they seek care. On the one hand, they appear able to decide for themselves; on the other hand, their parents remain legally responsible for them. Legal authorities conclude that the physician may respond to their requests under the following conditions: (1) The patient is at the age of discretion (15 years or older) and appears able to understand the procedure and its risks sufficiently to be able to give a genuinely informed consent; (2) the medical measures are taken for the patient's own benefit (i.e., not as a transplant donor or research subject); (3) the measures can be justified as necessary by medical opinion; and (4) there is some good reason, including simple refusal by the minor to request it, why parental consent cannot be obtained. It is also advisable for the physician to clarify with the minor any billing arrangements, since medical bills sent to parents may breach the confidentiality of the patient.

Benatar D. Non-therapeutic pediatric interventions. In: Singer PA, Viens AM, eds. *Cambridge Textbook of Biomedical Ethics*. New York, NY: Cambridge University Press: 2008:127–132.

Kenny N, Downie J, Harrison C. Respectful involvement of children in medical decision making;sIn: Singer PA, Viens AM, eds. *Cambridge Textbook of Biomedical Ethics*. New York, NY: Cambridge University Press: 2008:121–126.

Miller R. Role responsibility in pediatrics: appeasing or transforming. In: Frankel LR, Goldworth A, Rorty MV, Silverman WA, eds. *Ethical Dilemmas in Pediatrics*. New York, NY: Cambridge University Press; 2005:21–29.

2.2P Parental Incapacity

Pediatricians and other providers may occasionally suspect parents of serious incompetence in the care of their child. This suspicion must be carefully evaluated. In some cases, a parent or parents may manifest the signs of a psychiatric disorder that might render them incapacitated for rational consideration of matters concerning their child. For example, Munchausen syndrome by proxy is sometimes encountered when parents covertly make their children ill. A psychiatrically disabled parent may constitute a danger to the child. The existence and extent of psychiatric disease should be evaluated and, if indicated, Child Protective Services should be notified. Another sort of incompetence is manifested by parents who seem unable to comprehend the needs and interests of a child. Failure to provide for the ordinary needs of a child may represent incompetence caused by ignorance, moral turpitude, or substance addiction. In other cases, failure may be due to parental inexperience or to social conditions. Suspicion of incompetence should be evaluated for its degree, causes, remediability, and so forth. Most important, the alleged incompetence should be relevant to the problem at hand. Social workers and others expert at evaluation of social and environmental conditions are invaluable contributors. If suspicions are verified, legal remedies may be sought depending on the seriousness and urgency of the situation.

Garcia-Cariega M, Kerner JA. Munchausen syndrome by proxy; Kamm FM. Some conceptual and ethical issues in Munchausen syndrome by proxy. In: Frankel LR, Goldworth A, Rorty MV, Silverman WA, eds. *Ethical Dilemmas in Pediatrics*. New York, NY: Cambridge University Press; 2005:55–66; 67–79.

Levi BH. Child abuse and neglect. In: Singer PA, Viens AM, eds. *The Cambridge Textbook in Bioethics*. New York, NY: Cambridge University Press; 2008:132–142.

2.3P *Standard for Parental Preferences*

When parents are properly identified and appear competent as decision makers, they are morally and legally required to observe certain standards in their decision for their child. In general, they must promote the best interests of the child. In pediatric care, the appropriate course of treatment will usually represent the pursuit of the child's interests: restoration of health, relief of pain, support of growth, etc. However, in some situations, the best interest of the child may be unclear. This happens when a decision about forgoing life-supporting or life-saving interventions must be made. What standards, then, must guide parental choice in this difficult matter? We offer the following considerations:

(a) A well-founded judgment of medical inefficacy or futility justifies a parental decision to discontinue treatment that is supporting the life of a child. However, physicians and parents may disagree about this judgment. Parents may too quickly reach a judgment of inefficacy when treatment does not produce an immediate result or, overcome by the frustration of a long illness, conclude that treatment is futile. More commonly, parents may be emotionally unable to acknowledge the failure of treatment to save their child. They may demand that "everything be done" to maintain the biological viability of the child even in circumstances where the physician regards further treatment as inefficacious or futile. The physician has the duty to educate the parents, to explain the medical situation, and to strive to achieve a common understanding. Naturally, every effort must be made to reach an amicable understanding. However, it must be clear that the physicians and the institution have no ethical obligation to continue to provide treatment that, in their best professional judgment, is inefficacious or futile (see Section 1.2.2).

(d) If intervention is not clearly ineffective or futile, decisions should be made in view of the best interests of the infant or child. The phrase "best interests" is explained in Sections 2.4 and 3.0.7. Here the interests of the decision makers, namely, the parents and the physicians, or the interests of society at large are not the central focus: The interests of the patient constitute the standard for decisions made by others on behalf of that patient.

(e) In cases where differences of opinion exist between parents and physicians or between parents themselves, a review by an ethics committee or an ethics consultation may be helpful. If differences are irreconcilable, it may be necessary in rare cases to have recourse to the legal system that has been established to protect the welfare of those incapable of protecting themselves. Such recourse is often extremely traumatic for all concerned, but it acknowledges that the infant or child, despite its inability to speak for itself, has a valued place in our society.

2.4P Refusal of Treatment by Minor Children on Grounds of Religious Belief

Children may sometimes refuse medical treatment because they belong to religious groups that repudiate medical care. This poses a difficult problem for physicians.

Freedom of religion is highly valued and is protected by the Constitution of the United States. However, it is the freedom of the believer, capable of free and informed adherence to a faith, that is valued. In the words of a Supreme Court decision about the authority of a Jehovah's Witness parent, "Parents may be free to become martyrs themselves, but it does not follow that they are free to make martyrs of their children" (*Prince v Massachusetts*, 1944).

Even so, parents are given some latitude in determining appropriate treatments for their children. In a 1991 case, the Delaware Supreme Court permitted the Christian Scientist parents of a 3-year-old child suffering from Burkitt's lymphoma to refuse chemotherapy that had a 40% chance of success. The court reasoned that the probability of success, when weighed against the parents' interests in directing the child's care and the possible harmful effects of the chemotherapy, was too low to justify forcing the child to undergo the medical treatment (*Newmark v Williams*, Delaware, 1991).

Even in states with religious exemptions, physicians and hospitals should be prepared to bring before the Child Protective Agency and to the courts any case involving "medical interventions of clear efficacy that can prevent, ameliorate, or cure serious disease, incapacity, or loss of life and interventions that will clearly result in prevention of future handicaps or disability for the child" (Child Abuse Prevention and Treatment Act, 1985, "Baby Doe Regulations").

American Academy of Pediatrics Committee on Bioethics. Religious objections to medical care. *Pediatrics.* 1997;99:279.

Quality of Life

Quality of life is the third topic that must be reviewed to analyze a problem in clinical ethics. The idea of quality of life is difficult to define. However, it is often raised in complex cases and must be addressed. This chapter is devoted to explaining the concept of quality of life, analyzing its implications for clinical decisions, and suggesting certain distinctions and cautions that should be observed in discussing this concept in clinical care. The chapter also reviews in detail an area of clinical care in which quality-of-life considerations often loom large, namely, end-of-life care, including termination of life-support and physician-assisted dying.

3.0.1 The Ethical Principle of Beneficence as Satisfaction

No single ethical principle predominates in this discussion of quality of life. Both principles that we have discussed in the prior topics, namely, Beneficence and Respect for Autonomy, are relevant to this topic. However, we may select one particular aspect of the Principle of Beneficence as most relevant to this discussion about Quality of Life. In Topic One, we limited the very broad idea of Beneficence to one of its implications, namely, as a moral principle that directs persons to help others in need. In medicine that need arises from deficits in health, and the actions are those that correct those deficits and support the patient. In this topic, we focus on another aspect of the Principle of Beneficence, namely, acting in ways that bring satisfaction to other persons. Many moral philosophers have taken satisfaction or happiness as a significant element of beneficence. We propose that it is particularly relevant to clinical decisions. One significant feature of all medical interventions is the aim to produce a state of satisfaction for the patient who has sought treatment. He or she is not only made well, but *feels* well. *Quality of life, then, refers to that degree of satisfaction that people experience and value about their lives as a whole, and in its particular aspects, such as physical health.* The ethical dimensions of any case in clinical medicine must include not only appropriateness of interventions (Beneficence as Help) and respect for the patient's preferences (Autonomy), but also the improvement of quality of life (Beneficence as Satisfaction). When medical care fails to do so, ethical problems will arise, as this topic will demonstrate.

Beauchamp TL, Childress JM. Utilitarianism. In: Beauchamp TL, Childress JF, eds. *Principles of Biomedical Ethics*. 6th ed. New York, NY: Oxford University Press; 2009:336–343.

3.0.2 Meaning of Quality of Life

When defined as a state of satisfaction, quality of life expresses a value judgment: the experience of living, as a whole or in some aspect, is judged to be good or bad, better or worse. In recent years, efforts have been made to develop measures of quality of life that can be used to give some empirical basis to this value judgment and to evaluate outcomes of clinical interventions. Such measures list a variety of physical functions, such as mobility, performance of activities of daily living, absence or presence of pain, social interaction, and mental acuity. Scales are devised to rate the range of performance and satisfaction with these aspects of living. These various measures attempt to provide an objective description of what is inevitably a highly subjective and personal evaluation. Empirical studies of this subject are difficult to design and are limited in application. Also, individuals may deviate, often in striking ways, from the general views described in empirical surveys. Taken in this more empirical sense, Quality of Life may be defined as a multidimensional construct that includes "performance and enjoyment of social roles, physical health, intellectual functioning, emotional state, and life satisfaction or well-being." (Pearlman RA, Uhlmann RF. Quality of life in the elderly. *J Appl Gerontol*. 1988;7(3):316–330.)

Some authors distinguish quality of life from sanctity of life. By the term *sanctity*, they mean that human life represents the highest value that must be strenuously protected and preserved. Some authors use this term to assert that physical life must be sustained under any conditions and for as long as possible. In this view, evaluations of quality of life are irrelevant if they lead to any diminution of efforts to sustain life. This view has deep roots in some religious traditions. It also has a secular counterpart called "vitalism" that is sometimes encountered in medicine: organic life must be preserved even when all other human functions are lost. It is our belief that the profound respect for human life expressed in the phrase "sanctity of life" is not incompatible with decisions to refrain from medical treatments that prolong life in the particular circumstances that will be stated within this Topic.

3.0.3 Examples of Quality-of-Life Considerations in Clinical Care

A fundamental goal of medical care is the improvement of the quality of life for those who need and seek care. All of the goals of medicine stated in Section 1.0.9, such as relief of pain and improvement of function, are related to this fundamental objective. Patients seek medical attention because they are distressed by symptoms, worried by doubts about their health, or disabled by accidents and disease. The physician responds by examining, evaluating, diagnosing, treating, curing, comforting, and educating. These activities aim at improvement of the quality of the patient's life.

The cases of four patients described in Section 1.0.8 illustrate how medical treatment may affect quality of life in various ways. Mr. Cure's headache, stiff neck, and malaise are symptoms of meningitis. These symptoms can be relieved by administering an antibiotic that will eliminate the infection causing them. The quality of his life, impaired by the infection, is rapidly restored to normal. In other situations, the quality of the patient's life is seriously disrupted by a disease for which no cure is available; the patient is permanently, or will become, progressively disabled. Medical intervention aims at reduction of discomfort and maintenance of normal functions to the extent possible. For example, the quality of life for Mr. Care who has multiple sclerosis, is generally diminished but made "tolerable" by various medical, nursing, and rehabilitative interventions. In other situations, a patient's disease may be treated by an intervention that may cure the disease or retard its progress but, at the same time, reduce the quality of the patient's life. For example, Ms. Cope, a patient with brittle diabetes, will have to endure a strict dietary and insulin regimen, and Ms. Comfort will have to undergo a mastectomy and multiple courses of chemotherapy and radiotherapy in the attempt to conquer her cancer.

These cases support our view that an essential component of good care is the improvement of the patient's quality of life. The evaluation of quality of life is always relevant to providing appropriate medical care. Patients and their physicians must determine what quality of life is desirable and attainable, how it is to be achieved, and what risks and disadvantages are associated with the desired quality. The risks and benefits of medical interventions are relatively immediate when aimed at the reversal of a curable disease process. The risks and benefits associated with quality of life also focus on the long-term consequences of accepting or refusing a recommendation for medical intervention. If the patient consents to treatment, what sort of life will the patient have during and after the treatment? These considerations should be part of all serious discussions of medical choices. However, they raise ethical questions in several ways: (1) when there is a notable divergence between quality of life as assessed by physicians and by patients, (2) when patients are unable to express their evaluation about the quality of life they are likely to experience, (3) when the enhancement of normal qualities is sought as a goal of medicine, (4) when quality of life seems to have been entirely lost, and (5) when quality of life is used as an objective standard for the distribution of scarce health care. The first four issues are discussed in this topic; the fifth is discussed in Topic Four.

We ask seven questions about how quality of life is relevant to the identification and assessment of any clinical ethical problem:

1. What are the prospects, with or without treatment, for a return to normal life, and what physical, mental, and social deficits might the patient experience even if treatment succeeds?
2. On what grounds can anyone judge that some quality of life would be undesirable for a patient who cannot make or express such a judgment?
3. Are there biases that might prejudice the provider's evaluation of the patient's quality of life?
4. What ethical issues arise concerning improving or enhancing a patient's quality of life?
5. Do quality-of-life assessments raise any questions regarding changes in treatment plans, such as forgoing life-sustaining treatment?
6. What are the plans and rationale to forgo life-sustaining treatment?
7. What is the legal and ethical status of suicide?

3.0.4 Question One—What are the Prospects, With or Without Treatment, for a Return to Normal Life, and What Physical, Mental, and Social Deficits Might the Patient Experience Even If Treatment Succeeds?

The term "normal life" defies any single definition. Quality-of-life judgments are not based on a single dimension, nor are they entirely subjective or objective. They must consider personal and social function and performance, symptoms, prognosis, and the often unique values that patients ascribe to the quality of their life. Several important questions must be addressed: (1) Who is making the evaluation—the person living the life or an observer? (2) What criteria are being used for evaluation? And finally, the crucial ethical question: (3) What types of clinical decisions are justified by reference to quality-of-life judgments?

3.0.5 Distinctions About Quality of Life

It is important to distinguish between two uses of the phrase *quality of life*. Failure to do so causes confusion in clinical discussions.

(a) *In its most proper meaning, "quality of life" refers to the personal satisfaction expressed or experienced by individuals about their own physical, mental, and social situation.* This personal evaluation of an individual's own quality of life is an essential component of patient preferences, as we have explained in Topic Two. In this sense, ethical decisions about quality of life are based upon the ethics of personal autonomy: people make and express their own evaluation of the quality of their own life.

EXAMPLE I. A 27-year-old gymnastics instructor who is paralyzed because of a cervical spinal cord lesion may say, "My life isn't as bad as it looks to you. I've come to terms with my loss and have discovered the joys of intellectual life."

EXAMPLE II. A 68-year-old artist who is a diabetic with a 30-year history of Type II diabetes now faces blindness and multiple amputations. She says, "I wonder if I can endure a life of such poor quality?"

(b) *The phrase "quality of life" may also refer to an observer's evaluation of someone else's experiences of personal life.* Quality of life, understood in this sense, produces many of the ethical problems explored in this chapter.

EXAMPLE III. A parent says of a 29-year-old cognitively impaired son with an IQ score of 40, "He used to seem so happy, but now he's become so restless and difficult. What kind of quality of life does he have?"

EXAMPLE IV. An 83-year-old woman with advanced dementia, who is bedridden and tube-fed, is described by the nurses as "having poor quality of life."

COMMENT. Reference to quality of life in a clinical discussion is natural and necessary but, because the phrase can be used in so many ways, its use can cause confusion. Several points may dispel the confusion.

(a) *The judgment of poor quality of life may be made by the one who lives the life (personal evaluation) or by an observer (observer evaluation).* It often happens that lives considered by observers to be of poor quality are considered satisfactory or at least tolerable by the one living that life. Human beings are amazingly adaptive. They can make the best of the options available. For example, the quadriplegic gymnastics instructor may be a person of extraordinary motivation; the blind artist may enjoy a vivid imagination; the developmentally disabled person may enjoy games and interaction with others. Thus, if patients are able to evaluate and express their own quality of life, observers should not presume to know or judge but should seek the patients' personal evaluation. Similarly, when the person's own evaluation is not or cannot be known, clinicians or others should be extremely cautious in applying their own values.

(b) *Poor quality of life might mean, in general, that the sufferer's experiences fall below some standard that the observer considers desirable.* The observer, for example, may highly prize intellectual life or athletic prowess. But in each case, the experience in question is different; it may be pain, loss of mobility, presence of multiple debilitating health problems, loss of mental capacity and of the enjoyment of human interaction, loss of joy in life, and so on. Each of these may have a different significance for the one who experiences them compared to an observer's evaluation.

(c) *Evaluation of the quality of life, like life itself, changes with time.* The artist's concern may be the result of a depression that will resolve as she discovers her future possibilities; the gymnastics instructor may later become deeply depressed. Often clinicians see a patient when their quality of life is most compromised by trauma or sickness. Neither patients nor clinicians should make momentous decisions on the basis of possibly transitory conditions.

(d) *The evaluation of observers may reflect bias and prejudice.* For example, opinion that persons with developmental disabilities have "poor quality of life," may reflect a cultural bias in favor of intelligence and productivity. Prejudice may incline some people to judge that persons of a certain ethnic origin, social status, or sexual preference cannot possibly have good quality of life. Such prejudices must be acknowledged and, particularly in clinical care, be overcome.

(e) *The evaluation of quality of life, both by the one experiencing it and by observers, may reflect socioeconomic conditions such as homelessness, unavailability of home care, of rehabilitation, or of special education.* These obstacles, while very real, can often be overcome by planning and effort on the part of those caring for such patients.

EXAMPLE. Dax Cowart, whose case is often described in bioethics courses, was very badly burned and sustained a long, painful treatment and rehabilitation. He believed that his disabilities caused by the explosion—blindness, disfigurement, and crippling—would make his life intolerable and not worth living. He refused treatment and wished to die. He personally assessed his future quality of life as not worth living. Later, Dax revised his earlier assessment as he gradually overcame depression. He learned to appreciate mental activities, to enjoy social interaction, and to cope with his frustrations. He became a lecturer about his own story and an advocate for patients' rights and personal autonomy. He graduated from law school, passed the bar, and practiced law. He deals daily with his disabilities, but he has achieved a quality of life that he could not previously have imagined (although he still believes that he should not have been deprived of the right to refuse treatment). In addition to Dax's personal assessment, the physicians, surgeons, and nurses who cared for him offered observer assessments that were more optimistic than Dax's. They had seen badly burned patients recover to an acceptable quality of life despite their disabilities. The story of Dax Cowart vividly portrays the importance of quality of life as well as the difficulty of applying differing and varying judgments of quality of life in clinical decision making.

Confronting death: Who chooses? Who decides? A dialogue between Dax Cowart and Robert Burt. *Hastings Cent Rep.* 1998;28(1):14–28.

3.0.6 Question Two—On What Grounds Can Anyone Judge that Some Quality of Life Would be Undesirable for a Patient Who Cannot Make or Express Such a Judgment?

The considerations stated under "Surrogate Decision making" in Section 2.4 are all relevant to this question. This sections explains that when no preferences of the patient are known, surrogate decision-makers are held to make judgments that serve "the best interests of the patient." This idea of "best interest" is particularly relevant to our topic of quality of life.

3.0.7 Best Interest Standard and Quality of Life

The concept of best interest is drawn from the law, where it is commonly applied in cases of child custody: Which arrangement will best foster the healthy maturing of the child? Application of the term is very difficult in clinical medicine, where it is most often encountered in surrogate decisions about seriously ill persons whose prospects for recovery to health are remote. The first step in understanding how to apply this complex concept is to reflect on the interests, which all humans seem to share. *It can be presumed that all humans have an interest in being alive, being capable of understanding and communicating their thoughts and feelings, being able to control and direct their lives, being free from pain and suffering, and being able to attain desired satisfactions.* It can be presumed that all humans would choose to avoid loss of these abilities. Best interests can be understood as the set of elements that make up quality of life, as we have described earlier (see Section 3.0.2).

These general presumptions must be adapted to individual cases. What counts as an interest should be designated, as much as possible, from the viewpoint of the one for whom the judgment is being made. The interests common to competent, mature persons may not even occur to persons who are immature or who have diminished understanding and judgment. Still, they have interests in personal values suited to their conditions. Surrogate decision-makers should attempt, as much as possible, to view the world through the eyes of such persons rather than their own. Each situation in which these presumptions are challenged calls for close ethical evaluation. Critical assessment also consists in scrutinizing socially shared values for prejudice, discrimination, misinformation, and stereotyping.

Beauchamp TL, Childress JF. The best interest standard. In: Beauchamp TL, Childress JF, eds. *Principles of Biomedical Ethics*. 6th ed. New York, NY: Oxford University Press; 2009:138–140.

3.1 DIVERGENT EVALUATIONS OF QUALITY OF LIFE

Because evaluation of quality of life is so subjective, observers will rate certain forms of living quite differently. This diversity gives rise to several common major problems in clinical ethics: (1) lack of understanding about the patient's own values, (2) divergence between physicians' assessment of their patients' quality of life and the assessments made by patients themselves, (3) bias and discrimination that negatively affect the physician's dedication to the patient's welfare, and (4) the introduction of social worth criteria into quality-of-life judgments.

Studies have shown that physicians consistently rate their patient's quality of life lower than do the patients themselves. In one study, physicians and patients were asked independently to evaluate living with certain chronic conditions, such as arthritis, ischemic heart disease, chronic pulmonary disease, and cancer. Physicians judged life with these conditions to be less tolerable than did the patients who suffered from them. Physicians based their assessments primarily on disease conditions, whereas patients took into account nonmedical factors, such as interpersonal relationships, finances, and social conditions. Also, studies have shown that clinicians' quality-of-life assessments strongly influence clinical decisions such as those about resuscitation or forgoing life-support.

EXAMPLE. A 62-year-old man who had a brainstem stroke is disoriented and incapacitated. He is also diagnosed with uremia, secondary to obstructive nephropathy. His physician believes that uremia is a peaceful way to die, because the disabilities from the stroke could be very distressing to the patient. The physician suggests to the patient's surrogate that it may be in the patient's best interest to forgo surgery to relieve the obstruction. The surrogate chooses surgical treatment. The patient recovers and lives an additional 10 months with a satisfactory quality of life until shortly before his death.

COMMENT. This sort of divergence in evaluation can lead to serious misjudgments about the appropriateness of therapy. It is essential that physicians discuss the issue of quality of life with the surrogate and attempt to determine as explicitly as possible the values held by the patient. They should also acknowledge that even though their evaluations may derive from long clinical experience, they also reflect personal values that might not be shared by the patient. The phrase "if this were me" (so called Golden Rule reasoning) fails to take into account the patient's values and thus is misleading. Physicians should determine the best interests of competent patients by discussing quality-of-life options with them. If patients are incompetent or lack decision-making capacity, discussions with authorized surrogates are essential.

3.1.1 Question Three—Are There Biases That Might Prejudice the Provider's Evaluation of the Patient's Quality of Life?

One of the important ethical tenets of medicine is that the sick should be cared for regardless of race, religion, gender, or nationality. Individual physicians, however, may have beliefs and values that lead to biased and discriminatory judgments against certain persons or classes of persons. These judgments may affect clinical decisions.

(a) *Racial Bias.* The history of American medicine is stained by discrimination against African Americans, Native Americans, and other ethnic groups. Today these biases may be less explicit but still present; many studies reveal that racial and cultural minorities receive lower quality of care. It is ethically important that these biases be identified and eliminated from clinical decisions. (Institute of Medicine. *Unequal Treatment: Confronting Racial and Ethnic Disparities in Health Care.* Washington, D.C., 2002. *www.iom.edu/reports*)

(b) *Bias against the Elderly and the Disabled.* Studies have revealed that many physicians, particularly younger ones, are biased against elderly and disabled patients. They are reluctant to deal with them and sometimes make prejudicial judgments about them.

CASE. A 92-year-old woman is brought unconscious to the emergency department (ED). On examination, she is unresponsive, dehydrated, and hypotensive. She is also found to have a urinary tract infection and pulmonary infiltrates, possibly caused by aspiration. The ED resident believes she has sepsis from a urinary tract source but wonders whether to start antibiotics and fluid resuscitation because of her advanced age. The attending physician orders treatment. On recovery, the patient returns to her previous rather vigorous and alert quality of life, which had not been known to the treating ED physicians.

COMMENT. Treatment decisions should be based on medical need and patient preferences. Discrimination against persons on the basis of their chronological age is ethically wrong. Chronological age is only relevant to a clinical decision when it figures in an evidence-based judgment about a patient's likely response to an intervention. For example, persons older than 75 years are generally not good candidates for organ transplantation because of comorbidities such as cardiovascular disease.

(c) *Lifestyle Bias*. Studies have revealed that physicians are no more free from prejudices than the general population. Lifestyles such as homelessness or homosexual identity, or diseases such as alcoholism and substance abuse evoke negative attitudes or discomfort. These biases may, at times, affect clinical judgment, even quite unconsciously.

(d) *Gender Bias*. Gender bias exists, overtly or covertly, throughout our society. In health care, studies demonstrate that male physicians discount women's health complaints and that research has been designed in ways that fail to appropriately evaluate treatments for women. Prejudices often discount the intelligence and autonomy of women. It is also possible that female physicians have stereotypical attitudes toward their patients—male or female.

(e) *Social Worth*. Quality of life can be confused with social worth, that is, judgments about the value of a person's contribution to society. *A social worth evaluation counts persons who are productive, prominent, engaged, and creative as being more valuable than persons who lack those characteristics.* While judgments of this sort may be necessary for many social functions, they have no place in clinical decisions. Clinicians should not provide differential care to persons of social worth because of their presumed contribution to society except in most unusual circumstances (e.g., giving priority to a wounded president before his or her aides). The social worth view is particularly problematic when decisions about scarce treatment, such as organ transplantation are at stake (see Section 4.5.5).

RECOMMENDATION. In general, social worth criteria are not relevant to diagnosis and treatment of patients. Quality of life is about a particular patient's life as they experience it, not about his or her social status, importance, or productivity. Patients should not be afforded or refused treatment on the basis of social worth. It is not the physician's prerogative to make such judgments in the context of providing medical treatment. Criminals, addicts, and terrorists should be treated in relation to their medical need, not their social worth. The special features of triage decisions will be treated in Section 4.5.3.

3.1.2 The Challenging Patient

In Section 2.5 several patients were described whose quality of life made it difficult to care for them. Ms. Cope was uncooperative, alcoholic, and unpleasant. Another patient was an abusive drug addict. Health care providers may find such patients exasperating, disagreeable, and even repugnant. This reaction may distort clinical decisions about such patients and affect the quality of care provided to them. Providers should make strenuous efforts to overcome their negative attitudes toward such patients.

EXAMPLE. Mr. C.D. is a homeless man who inhabits building excavations. He is filthy, foul mouthed, and, at times, violent and disruptive. He appears quite regularly at the hospital in need of various sorts of care for pneumonia, frostbite, delirium tremens, and so forth. He is brought to the ED for the second time in a month with bleeding esophageal varices. At morning report, one of the house officers asks whether Mr. C.D.'s quality of life should disqualify him from treatment.

COMMENT. Mr. C.D.'s lifestyle should not preclude physicians from attending to his medical needs. Particular aspects of that lifestyle, such as ability to follow a treatment regimen should be taken into consideration in developing a treatment plan. He does, however, impose certain burdens on his providers and on society that may be relevant to judgments about his care. This contextual factor is considered in Topic Four.

3.1.3 Developmental Disability

Persons whose aptitudes are limited as a result of developmental or cognitive disability are often objects of discrimination. Given the range of possibilities for social intercourse, intellectual achievement, personal accomplishment, and productivity open to most human beings, the lives of these persons may seem severely restricted and their lives can be described as different in quality from those without those disabilities. When decisions about medical care are made for such persons, is such a different quality of life ever a relevant consideration?

EXAMPLE. Joseph Saikewicz was a 67-year-old man who had been institutionalized for severe developmental disability since he was 1 year old. His mental age was estimated at less than the 3-year-old level, and his IQ score was recorded as 10. He develops acute myelogenous leukemia. His guardian says, "His life is of such poor quality. Why should we try to extend it?"

COMMENT. The Massachusetts Supreme Court approved (after his death) a decision not to treat Joseph Saikewicz with chemotherapy. The court attempted to distinguish between general quality of life of developmentally disabled persons, which it did not consider relevant, and the specific quality of life that Joseph Saikewicz "was likely to experience" if he had been treated with chemotherapy. Speaking of the continued state of pain and disorientation likely to result from chemotherapy, the court said, "he would have experienced fear without the understanding from which other patients draw strength." This distinction suggests a point of ethical importance. It directs attention to the quality of life as experienced by the patient and away from the quality of life typical of persons with profound mental disability. It is ethically dangerous to decide to withhold medical treatment from an individual because that individual belongs to a class of disabled persons. Such decisions look more to the burden these persons place on society than to the burden these persons themselves experience. Seeing persons only as class members for the purpose of medical treatment starts a process in which classes of "undesirables" grow increasingly wider and include more and more persons who are "burdens to themselves and others." This can lead to invidious discrimination. Quality-of-life assessments should focus on the quality of the life being lived by a particular patient.

3.1.4 Dementia and Quality of Life

The occurrence of Alzheimer's disease (AD) or any other dementing disease is a tragedy for patients and families. These medical conditions entail serious deterioration in quality of life as perceived by the patient and by others. They pose challenges to health care practitioners. Some of those challenges are ethical in nature: truthfully informing the patient of the diagnosis as well as imposing limits on lifestyle, such as driving, deciding about living arrangements, use of restraints, and treatment at the end of life. In recent years, improvements in the understanding of these conditions and in treatment of persons suffering from them have alleviated some burdens. In general, the ethical approach to such conditions calls for the least restrictive measures compatible with the safety and comfort of the patient. In addition, other ethical problems may arise.

CASE. Mr. R.P., an accomplished cabinetmaker and a congenial, loving person, begins to show the characteristic signs of AD at the age of 66. He slips rapidly into extreme forgetfulness and confusion, accompanied by outbreaks of anger, particularly at his wife of 40 years. His physician performs tests to exclude other possible causes. His sons, who are partners in his business, find it necessary to prevent him from coming to the factory and from entering his home workshop, which infuriates him. His physician treats him with donepezil and later adds memantine to control violent outbursts.

COMMENT. Although particular ethical quandaries are posed by patients with AD, the most general problem is the maintenance of their dignity, independence, sense of self-respect, and connection with their social and physical environment. These qualities are often seriously undermined by well-meaning care providers and by restrictive arrangements that often exacerbate the problems (e.g., restraints have been shown to accelerate physical and psychologic deterioration and to increase sedative drug use). Many techniques have been devised to support the dignity of even badly affected patients and have been shown to improve their quality of life; advice from clinicians experienced in the care of such patients is helpful. Medication may have positive effects on some problems commonly associated with AD, such as depression, delusions, and aggressive behavior. However, no drug treatment has yet been shown to restore lost cognitive function.

RECOMMENDATION. In Mr. R.P.'s case, use of donepezil and memantine may have some positive effect because its efficacy appears to be greatest in stabilizing the condition in earlier stages of AD. However, this effect generally is not lasting, and the patient will return to progressive dementia. Thus, providers and family should seriously consider whether a transitory and slight improvement in mental status will truly improve the patient's quality of life. The patient will again slip into dementia, repeating the distressing experience of loss of capacity. Also, antidementia medicines may have unpleasant side effects, such as nausea, diarrhea, and insomnia that might be particularly distressing to a person with diminished mental function. This medical intervention that, in principle, may be medically indicated, as well as desired by the surrogates, may have a detrimental effect on the overall quality of life of the patient. In this sense, then, quality of life, in the sense of producing satisfaction, does become a relevant ethical consideration.

3.1.5 Question Four—What Ethical Issues Arise Concerning Improving or Enhancing a Patient's Quality of Life?

Medicine improves quality of life by remedying the effects of illness. We call attention to four areas of medicine in which efforts to improve quality of life raise ethical issues: (1) rehabilitation, (2) palliative care, (3) treatment of chronic pain, and (4) enhancement.

3.1.6 Rehabilitation Ethics

Rehabilitation medicine aims to improve quality of life, as demonstrated by restoration of mobility, ability to work, and independent living. The autonomy of the patient is a primary goal, and the preferences and values of the patient define the goal. The cooperation of the patient is crucial. In this setting, several special ethical problems predominate. These problems sometimes arise because the patient's preferences and judgment of personal quality of life may conflict with the physiatrist's medical knowledge and values.

EXAMPLE. A program of rehabilitation is recommended to the gymnastics instructor described in Section 3.0.5. He initially refuses to participate, stating, "I'm crippled and the quality of my life is so bad that it can't be improved." The rehabilitation team has a different view of his possibilities. They invite him to continue to discuss the issues and they propose some short-term goals.

COMMENT. This case could be discussed in Topic Two, because it is an instance of problems arising around patient preferences. However, quality of life is central, to the physiatrist's evaluation of whether the patient's wishes should be honored. Rehabilitation medicine stresses an educational framework for treatment: persons are taught skills and taught to live within the limits of inevitable disabilities. In this case, the principal problem is not the physical one of improving mobility. It is the educational problem of leading this patient to a different perception of the quality of his life, in which he can find full satisfaction.

3.1.7 Palliative Care and Treatment of Pain

Palliative care medicine is defined as "an approach that improves the quality of life of patients and their families facing the problems associated with life-threatening illness, through the prevention and relief of suffering by means of early identification, assessment, and treatment of pain and other problems, physical, psychosocial, and spiritual." (*World Health Organization*). Relief of pain is a traditional medical goal sought by medication, surgery, and physical therapy. However, concentration on the physiologic components of pain through pharmacologic or surgical interventions, without equal attention to the psychologic, social, and spiritual, may bring little relief. Even if relief is achieved in the physiologic sense, other important ethical responsibilities may be left unfulfilled; for example, aiding patients to deal with their impending death and its effect on others. Palliative care medicine utilizes methods to achieve these global aims. Physicians should make themselves aware of these components and seek assistance from palliative care specialists.

Many hospitals have established palliative care services. It is not uncommon for palliative care to be called into cases where there are ethical problems. Similarly, ethical consultation may be called in cases where palliative care is an issue. Very commonly, a palliative care referral occurs immediately after an ethical decision has been made to shift from intensive to comfort care. Possibly the patient's experiences and the family's agonies could have been alleviated if palliative care medicine had been involved before the critical decision to forgo life-sustaining treatment was made. Similarly, an earlier involvement of clinical ethics may facilitate the decision making, and suggest an earlier involvement of palliative care. Therefore, these two clinical specialties, palliative care and clinical ethics, must recognize their distinct competencies and collaborate in optimizing the care of the patient.

3.1.8 Treatment of Chronic Pain

Pain relief, like all other medical interventions, should be based on medical indications and on patient preferences. However, pain relief poses particular problems. Objective physical causes of pain are often difficult to discern. Yet, patients complain of pain without apparent physical cause. Care of these patients can be difficult.

CASE. Mr. T.W., a 42-year-old insurance broker, visits his physician, complaining of severe, diffuse pain, which, he said, had been "creeping up" on him for several months. Now, it is incessant and moves about the body, from upper back and shoulders to lower back and lower limbs. Standing for any length of time is excruciating. His physician does a thorough physical examination, prescribes several imaging tests, and, after negative results, recommends a neurology consultation, which is also unproductive. A variety of pain medications are prescribed, with little relief. Mr. T.W.'s pain continues to the point of disability. The physician finally tells him frankly, "We can't find anything wrong with you. Your pain is psychogenic; that is, it comes from the mind, not the body. You really should see a psychiatrist."

COMMENT. Chronic pain often poses a difficult medical problem because the specific organic cause is elusive. It also poses an ethical problem because many physicians, once they suspect a psychogenic origin, tend to dismiss the patient as a "somatizer." Patients will interpret comments such as that of the doctor in this case as an accusation that their pain is unreal or imagined. Even when a significant psychogenic component to pain is present, the pain is real. Instead of dismissing the patient with such a remark, physicians should provide symptomatic relief and consult with experts in pain management and in physical medicine. Psychologic assistance should be recommended as assistance in coping with pain, rather than as a substitute for medical management. If the patient requests certification for Workman's compensation, the physician should respond truthfully. If, after adequate workup and appropriate therapeutic efforts, complaints of pain persist and, if the physician has no well-grounded suspicion of malingering, it can be truly said that the patient experiences chronic, disabling pain. The forms that must be filled out for certification sometimes make it difficult to express the truth since they often require evidence of a physical cause for pain. In filling out such forms, physicians should provide honest and thorough clinical information.

3.2 ENHANCEMENT MEDICINE

Medical skills, traditionally devoted to the remedy of illness, are increasingly employed to improve normal conditions: cosmetic surgery responds to the desires of individuals for a more attractive appearance; administration of growth hormone increases height for short-statured persons; drugs improve sexual potency and mental acuity; and steroids augment athletic prowess. How do these enhancement capabilities fit the goals of medicine? Do they raise any special ethical problems for the clinician? Discussions of this issue often distinguish between treatment and enhancement. Treatments attempt to respond to physical, physiological, or psychological defects that deprive persons of normal characteristics. Enhancements augment already normal characteristics beyond the normal range. Because the meaning of "normal" in these descriptions is ambiguous, it is difficult to draw a sharp distinction between these two capabilities of medicine, as well as difficult to discern implications for the ethical responsibilities of physicians.

Treatments, however, remain closer to the usual procedures of medicine in that they are initiated because of an obvious deficit. For example, growth hormone is prescribed to augment a clinically proven growth hormone deficiency. Enhancements, on the other hand, do not remedy a documented physical or psychological deficit but respond to the desire of the patient (or sometimes their surrogates, as when parents request growth hormone for their short-statured children).

The desire for enhancements may stem from several motives, such as attaining competitive advantage, improving self-image and self-esteem, or feeling equal in one's peer group. These forms of enhancement raise questions about whether or not medical indications are present. Multiple ethical questions can be raised: do enhancements create unfairness in distribution of resources (competitive advantage goes to those able to afford enhancement), complicity with suspect cultural norms (idealized body types), interference with social practices (fairness in athletic competition), inauthenticity and false self-images? Some judge that enhancement medicine is little more than a lucrative commercial activity for the enrichment of practitioners. Others argue that the psychological benefits to patients may significantly improve their quality of life. The ethical questions raised by these practices are currently much debated. Thus, although many enhancement practices have entered into the daily practice of medicine, such as cosmetic surgery or the prescription of drugs for sexual potency, practitioners should be aware that many enhancement practices are on the fringe of the traditional goals of medicine and may have negative personal and social consequences.

Murray T. Enhancement. In: Steinbock B, ed. *The Oxford Handbook of Bioethics*. New York, NY: Oxford University Press; 2007:chap 21.

Parens E, ed. *Enhancing Human Traits: Conceptual Complexity and Ethical Implications*. Washington, DC: Georgetown University Press; 1998.

3.3 COMPROMISED QUALITY OF LIFE AND LIFE-SUSTAINING INTERVENTIONS

Questions about quality of life are often raised at times when patients are seriously ill and receiving intensive life-sustaining treatments. It is important to appreciate the relationship between quality-of-life evaluation and considerations about the use of life-sustaining treatment.

3.3.1 Question Five—Do Quality-of-Life Assessments Raise Any Questions Regarding Changes in Treatment Plans, Such as Forgoing Life-Sustaining Treatment?

Quality of life can be compromised in various ways. For purposes of description, we propose terms to describe three different ways in which compromised quality of life appears in clinical ethics considerations: restricted, severely diminished, and profoundly diminished. Each of these has implications for clinical decisions.

(a) *Restricted quality of life describes a situation in which a person suffers from severe deficits of physical or mental health.* Their ability to perform one or more common human activities is restricted by those deficits. In the presence of such restriction, the one who has the deficits, or observers, form an opinion about the worth of a life restricted in that manner. Clearly, as noted previously, opinions of the person living that life may differ significantly from the opinions of the observers. Persons such as amputees, paraplegics, those with learning disabilities, etc., commonly consider that they have a good quality of life, despite the deficits. It is one of the goals of medicine to support and enhance restricted quality of life

EXAMPLE. Ms. Cope, the diabetic patient who has multiple medical problems, considers her life, although restricted, to be valuable and worthwhile, whereas some observers may judge otherwise.

(b) *Severely diminished quality of life describes a form of life in which a person's general physical condition has seriously and irreversibly deteriorated, whose range of function is greatly limited, whose ability to communicate with others is minimal, and who may be suffering discomfort and pain.*

EXAMPLE. A very demented 85-year-old man is confined to bed with severe arthritis, persistent decubitus ulcers, and diminished respiratory capacity. He must be fed by tube and requires heavy pain medication.

COMMENT. This description differs from the former (a) in that the patient, while still sentient and reactive, has essentially lost the ability to communicate any personal evaluation of his or her experiences. The experiences are, to an observer, those that most persons would consider undesirable and wish to avoid. Also, we use the word "diminished" rather than "restricted" because, for the most part, in restricted situations, the patient can be an active participant, while in "diminished" situations, patients are hardly capable of active participation.

(c) *Profoundly diminished quality of life is an appropriate objective description of the situation in which the patient suffers extreme physical debilitation together with apparently complete and irreversible loss of sensory and intellectual activity.*

EXAMPLE. Mr. Care suffers an anoxic episode of 15 minutes after cardiopulmonary arrest. After 3 weeks, he has still not recovered consciousness. Physicians believe he is in a vegetative state.

COMMENT. This classification of quality of life describes a situation in which not only communicative abilities are lost but also the neurological capacities to process sensory input and mental activities. We use the term "profoundly" to indicate a deep and enduring loss. In this situation, only the observers' opinions contribute to deliberation about the value of such a state (absent some prior expression by the patient). Some observers believe that there is no quality of life, because the patient is incapable of the neural activities that generate satisfaction; other observers maintain that life as such, regardless of quality, is to be valued. These considerations are relevant to the clinical diagnosis of vegetative state, which we will discuss in Section 3.3.3.

We note that most persons, if given the choice, seem to consider severely (b) or profoundly diminished (c) quality of life undesirable. Studies suggest that most persons, when asked their opinions about such conditions, view them as "life not worth living" or "life worse than death." Thus, absent actual evidence of personal opinion to the contrary, it is not unreasonable to judge (b) and (c) as objectively undesirable. This is a cautious assumption, because studies suggest that persons often decide differently when imagining a situation than when they are actually in such a situation. Further, we do not take this assumption alone as the basis for any decision that would lead to termination of treatment and the death of the patient. The conditions explained in Topics One, Two, and Four must also be weighed in making a decision about what constitutes proportionate treatment (see Section 3.3.5).

Patrick DL, Pearlman RA, Starks HE, et al. Validation of preferences for life-sustaining treatment: implications for advance care planning. *Ann Intern Med.* 1997;127:509–517.

3.3.2 Severely Diminished Quality of Life

Patients whose condition fits the criteria for severely diminished quality of life may need life-sustaining interventions. The ethical question is whether the fact that the patient has a severely diminished quality of life makes it ethically permissible to discontinue life-supporting interventions.

CASE I. Mrs. A.W., a 34-year-old woman, married with three children, has had a history of scleroderma and ischemic ulcerations of fingers and toes. She is admitted to the hospital for treatment of renal failure. The big toe of her right foot and several fingers of her left hand became gangrenous. Several days later she consents to amputation of the right foot and the thumb and first finger of her left hand. After surgery, she is alternately obtunded and confused. She develops pneumonia and is placed on a respirator. The remaining fingers of her left hand become gangrenous, and more extensive amputation is required. Her renal condition worsens, and it is now necessary to consider initiating dialysis. The attending physician says, "How could anyone want to live a life of such terrible quality?" He asks himself whether dialysis should be withheld and whether the respirator should be discontinued.

CASE II. Mr. B.R. is an 84-year-old man living in a nursing home. He was diagnosed as having Alzheimer's dementia 5 years ago. He is wheelchair bound and does not respond meaningfully to human attention. He is often very agitated. He cannot now express, nor has he previously expressed, preferences regarding care. He is otherwise physically healthy. He is difficult to feed, frequently choking and expelling food. He has been treated several times in the past month for aspiration pneumonia with antibiotics and fluids. During the night, he develops a violent cough and wheezing. He has a fever of 100°F. The visiting physician diagnoses aspiration pneumonia. Should he be transferred to the hospital and treated?

CASE III. Robert Wendland suffered serious brain injury after rolling his truck at high speed. He remained in coma for 16 months before regaining consciousness. After 6 months of rehabilitation, Robert remained severely cognitively impaired, emotionally volatile, and physically handicapped. He was able to respond to simple commands, communicate inconsistently on a yes/no board, and engage in simple physical movements, such as drawing circles and a capital "R." While he could respond to simple questions, he did not answer the question whether he wished to die. A consulting neurologist described his condition as "a minimally conscious state ... [with] some cognitive function" and the ability to "respond to his environment," but not to "interact" with it "in a more proactive way." Robert required feeding by a jejunostomy tube. After the tube dislodged and was replaced three times, his wife refused to consent to further surgical intervention. Physicians agreed, as did the ethics committee. Robert's mother and sister insisted that treatment be continued.

COMMENT. In Case I of Mrs. A.W., the severe physical deficits and problems of rehabilitation faced by her, evoke in the observer an assessment that "No one would want to live that way." This, of course, cannot be verified by Mrs. A.W. at this time. She has a progressive disease with its associated problems. Many of these problems are susceptible to effective medical treatment and rehabilitation. In addition, she herself has consented to the initial amputations, suggesting her willingness to live with these deficits. Finally, her vital personality before her surgery suggested to the staff that she had the ability to cope with rehabilitation and the difficulties of subsequent life. Even though, at the time of her hospitalization, she seems to some observers to have severely diminished quality of life, Mrs A.W. should be viewed as a person with restricted quality of life.

In Case II that of Mr. B.R., nothing is known about how or whether he evaluates the quality of his life. Any judgment that his quality of life is severely restricted reflects an observer's assessment of the physical facts as well as an evaluation of living with extreme limitations of physical and mental activity and the painful and intrusive interventions needed to sustain physiological functions. If Mr. B.R.'s life continues, it is likely to deteriorate even further. He will probably suffer recurring episodes of aspiration. Quality of life, then, becomes a relevant ethical consideration. Is it ethically appropriate to assert that further supportive treatment is not in Mr. B.R.'s best interests?

Case III is an actual case decided by the *California Supreme Court* (Wendland, 2001). Mr. Robert Wendland's condition was diagnosed as "minimal consciousness." This recent diagnostic term describes persons with severe alterations in consciousness who do not meet diagnostic criteria for coma or for vegetative state. This condition ranges from awareness with an intermittent ability to communicate in limited ways to a near vegetative state with little awareness and virtually no ability to communicate. This state falls under our definition of severely restricted quality of life. A reasonable person may choose not to live such a life. However, in the absence of sufficient evidence that this patient would so judge, observers (physicians, surrogates, and family) cannot decide whether it is a life not worth living.

RECOMMENDATION. In Case I, it is ethically obligatory to continue to treat Mrs. A.W. Significant medical goals can still be attained and, although her current preferences cannot be ascertained, it can be presumed that she favors continued treatment. Many persons do live successfully and happily with such severe restrictions. She will have a restricted quality of life but not a severely or profoundly diminished one. The assumption that no rational person would desire to live in this state, justified in Mr. B.R.'s case, is not justified in the case of Mrs. A.W.

In Mr. B.R.'s case, it is ethically permissible to refrain from treating Mr. B.R.'s pneumonia after several episodes have shown this to be the beginning of an unpreventable recurring pattern. Tube feeding has risks of aspiration and infection. Also, clinical evidence reveals that patients with advanced dementia who are tube fed have neither any better nutritional status nor any longer survival than patients without tube feeding. A decision to forgo artificial nutrition and hydration can be justified on the basis of probabilistic futility (see Section 1.2.2), However, severely diminished quality of life is also a significant justification for these clinical decisions. There is no obligation to assist in sustaining a form of living that offers no perceptible satisfaction but only distress and suffering. It can be assumed that a rational person would not chose such a life.

In Case III, we believe that it is obligatory to sustain Mr. Robert Wendland, absent any clear evidence of his own preferences. The California Supreme Court did not authorize the conservator to deny surgical replacement of the feeding tube. (Mr. Wendland died before the decision was rendered.) Severely diminished quality of life, in itself, is not a sufficient reason to forgo life support; there must also be clear evidence, such as a written advance directive, of the patient's preferences.

3.3.3 Profoundly Diminished Quality of Life

Profoundly diminished quality of life is our designation of a situation in which the patient suffers extreme physical debilitation and complete and irreversible loss of sensory and intellectual activity. By definition, this judgment cannot result from personal evaluation, because any person in such a situation lacks the ability to perceive, understand, and evaluate his or her state.

CASE. Mr. Care, the patient with multiple sclerosis, is living at home. He has a respiratory arrest associated with gram-negative pneumonia and septicemia. He suffers approximately 15 minutes of anoxia before the arrival of emergency services. He is resuscitated, rushed to the hospital, and placed on a respirator. After 3 weeks, Mr. Care has not recovered consciousness and remains dependent on the respirator. A neurology consultant states that Mr. Care has the neurologic signs consistent with the vegetative state and that, while there is some remote chance of a very limited recovery, he believes that Mr. Care is highly likely to remain in a vegetative state. Mr. Care's family desire that weaning from the respirator be attempted. He is successfully weaned and, after several months, neurology affirms that he is still in a vegetative state. At no time in the course of his care has he expressed any clear preferences about his future. Should respiratory support be continued?

COMMENT.

(a) Mr. Care is not dead according to brain function criteria. That is, although he has lost, apparently permanently, most cortical functions, he still has brainstem activity, respiration, heartbeat and many spinal reflexes. Therefore, he is not legally dead (see Section 1.5).

(b) The diagnostic term "vegetative state" must be used with care, particularly when the words "persistent" or "permanent" are associated with it. Current usage recommends that the phrase "vegetative state" be applied to a neurological condition following severe head trauma or anoxic insult. The patient comes out of initial coma but shows no signs of consciousness of world or self. Persons in vegetative state retain hypothalamic and brainstem function, as well as spinal and cranial nerve reflexes. Their clinical appearance shows eye movement (but seldom tracking), pupillary adjustment to light, gag and cough reflex, movement of trunk and limbs. These patients also go through sleep–wake cycles, sometimes grimace, grin, groan, seem to weep and utter unintelligible articulations.

This condition can be called *continued vegetative state* if it persists for several months (the term "persistent" is no longer favored). Some neurologists use the term *"permanent" vegetative state* when it is judged to be irreversible. Permanent vegetative state is a neurologic prognosis defined as "a sustained, complete loss of self-aware cognition with wake/sleep cycles and other autonomic functions remaining relatively intact. The condition can either follow acute, severe bilateral cerebral damage or develop gradually as the end stage of a progressive dementia" (Jennett, 2002). A prognosis that the vegetative state is permanent can be reliably made after 3 months for anoxic insult and 1 year after trauma. The majority of these patients do not require respiratory support but do require artificial nutrition. Other neurologists reject the use of the term permanent vegetative state because it implies prognostic certainty inconsistent with a few but well-documented cases of late recovery of consciousness from a vegetative state.

The clinical signs of vegetative state, particularly, open eyes, limb movement, yawning and sleep–wake cycles lead observers, particularly family, to interpret these non-cognitive behaviors as signs of consciousness. Since these signs persist after the diagnosis of vegetative state, family members are sometimes confused about the prospects for the patient's recovery.

A further complicating factor is that some patients do recover consciousness from a vegetative state. The clinical diagnosis of "minimal consciousness" is made when there is intermittent evidence of self or environmental awareness, verbalization or simple but reproducible responses to commands or questions. Nevertheless, patients who display minimal consciousness remain significantly compromised and severely disabled. Although therapeutic and rehabilitative research is ongoing, little is know about how to effectively treat this condition. The case of Robert Wendland illustrates the confusion and controversy about minimal consciousness.

(c) Care must be taken not to mistake a vegetative state for another neurologic condition known as "locked-in state." In this latter condition, lesions in the midbrain paralyze efferent pathways governing movement and communication but leave consciousness intact. Neurologic consultation is required to make a differential diagnosis.

Giacino JT, Ashwal S, Childs N, et al. The minimally conscious state: definition and diagnostic criteria. *Neurology.* 2002;58(3):349–353.

Jennett B. *The Vegetative State: Medical Facts, Legal and Ethical Dilemmas.* New York, NY: Cambridge University Press; 2002.

Lo B. The persistent vegetative state. In: Lo B, ed. *Resolving Ethical Dilemmas: A Guide for Clinicians.* 4th ed. Philadelphia, PA: Lippincott Williams & Wilkins; 2009:162–165.

Medical aspects of the persistent vegetative state–first of two parts. The Multi-Society Task Force on PVS. *N Engl J Med.* 1995;330(21):1499–1508.

Medical aspects of the persistent vegetative state–second of two parts. The Multi-Society Task Force on PVS. *N Engl J Med.* 1995;330(22):1572–1579.

COMMENT. Compare this version of Mr. Care's case with Ms. Care's condition as described in Section 1.1.2. where his death is imminent. In that situation, the judgment that further intervention will not achieve any medical goals justifies the decision to discontinue mechanical support. This judgment is based upon probabilistic futility. In this present version of the case, Mr. Care is neither dead nor imminently dying. If his pneumonia resolves and he can be weaned from the respirator, he will not recover from his underlying disease, nor is he likely to return to mental functioning sufficient for consciousness and communication. On the other hand, if respirator support is removed, Mr. Care may breathe on his own and continue to live in a vegetative state. Life in a vegetative state seems to the physician and the family a life of very poor or of no quality. Their hope is that, once the respirator is discontinued, Mr. Care will die quickly.

RECOMMENDATION. In our judgment, it is ethically permissible to discontinue respiratory support and all other forms of life-sustaining treatment. This recommendation should be made to the family and their agreement secured. If they do not agree, the hospital's policy on nonbeneficial treatment should be invoked (see Section 1.2.2) We argue that the conjunction of three features of this case justifies such a decision:

(a) No goals of medicine other than support of organic life are being or will be accomplished. We do not believe that this goal alone is an overriding and independent goal of medicine.
(b) No preferences of the patient are known that might contradict the assumption that she would wish medical support for organic life discontinued. Usually, a judgment of the patient's best interests would substitute for their preferences. However, in the state of apparently irreversible loss of cognitive and communicative function, the individual no longer has any personal "interests," that is, nothing that happens to the patient can in any way advance his or her welfare nor can the individual evaluate any event or circumstances. If no interests can be served, life-sustaining interventions are not mandatory.
(c) The patient no longer has the neurologic/experiential capacities to feel satisfaction (or dissatisfaction) with his or her state. The essential element of qualify of life, namely, satisfaction, is lacking.
(d) The conjunction of these three ethical arguments (drawn from Topic One, "Medical Indications," Topic Two, "Patient Preferences," and Topic Three, "Quality of Life") justify the conclusion that physicians have no ethical obligation to continue life-sustaining interventions. When no interests of the patient are served, no medical goal other than sustaining organic life is achievable and there is no evidence that the patient would choose continued life, no duty to continue medical support exists. There may be other reasons, such as desire of family to see their loved one, that might justify continued support for a limited time.

CASE (CONTINUED). While Mr. Care is in a continuing vegetative state, he becomes anuric and is in renal failure. Should dialysis be initiated?

COMMENT.

(a) This version of the case involves an instance of not starting an intervention rather than stopping one already being used. Many interventions are initiated at times when their use is clearly indicated. The achievement of important goals is still seen as possible. When these goals cannot be achieved, and when there are other important considerations, for example, absence of patient preference and severely diminished quality of life, interventions may be discontinued. There is no ethical difference between starting or stopping an intervention in these circumstances.

(b) There may be emotional differences between starting and stopping treatment. Some physicians find it more troubling to stop an ongoing intervention than not to initiate a new one. The initiation of treatment may sustain some measure of hope. If, despite the physician's efforts, the patient succumbs to the disease, the physician has tried and done his or her best. Also, in withdrawing treatment, the physicians may feel responsible (in a causal sense) for the events that follow, even though they bear no responsibility (in the sense of ethical or legal accountability) either for the disease process or for the patient succumbing to the disease. These personal feelings, strong though they may be, do not alter the ethical judgment that, in these clinical situations, it is appropriate to refrain from initiating an intervention and also appropriate to discontinue it.

(c) Finally, after deciding to refrain from aggressive therapeutic efforts, new medical problems, such as infection or renal failure, sometimes tempt physicians to initiate therapeutic interventions to deal with these emergent problems. This is, of course, irrational, unless the intervention has as its purpose another goal more appropriate to the situation, such as providing comfort to the dying patient.

(d) The terminology, "Do Not Escalate" (DNE) is coming into use. This is a clinical order that further therapeutic measures to counter newly emergent clinical problems are not indicated. Current therapeutic, supportive, and palliative measures may be continued. If this terminology is used, it should be clearly defined and the rationale clearly stated.

RECOMMENDATION. The decision to forgo support is justified in both versions of Mr. Care's case. It is the common position of medical ethicists, supported by many judicial decisions, that the distinction between stopping and starting is neither ethically nor legally relevant. It is our position that there is no significant ethical difference between stopping and starting if the essential considerations regarding medical indications, patient preference, and quality of life are the same.

3.3.4 Artificially Administered Nutrition and Hydration

Artificially administered nutrition and hydration refers to a liquid preparation of calories, proteins, carbohydrates, fats, and minerals that are administered to the patient by means of a nasogastric or gastrostomy tube in order to sustain metabolic function when a patient is unable to take solid or liquid nutrition by mouth. It is used to feed patients with head and neck cancers or gastrointestinal disorders, after certain surgical procedures as well as patients who are comatose, demented, or in vegetative state.

CASES. Mr. Care has been started on intravenous fluids and nutrients while in coma after his respiratory arrest. Is it permissible to discontinue these measures after he is judged to be in permanent vegetative state? Mr. B.R. has deteriorated mentally and now lies in a fetal position, showing no response to verbal or tactile stimuli. Should a feeding tube be employed? In both cases, death would ensue from starvation and dehydration unless administered nutrients and fluids are used. Is there any special obligation to use these measures that distinguishes them from respiratory support, dialysis, or medication that can be ethically forgone?

Lo B. Tube and intravenous feedings. In: Lo B, ed. *Resolving Ethical Dilemmas: A Guide for Clinicians*. 4th ed. Philadelphia, PA: Lippincott Williams & Wilkins; 2009:145–150.

COMMENT. There has been considerable debate about this issue. Some authors argue that feeding is so basic a human function and so symbolic of care that it should never be forgone. They also note that forgoing these techniques is a direct cause of death by starvation. They wonder about the social implications of a policy that would deprive the most helpless of basic human attention. Other ethicists judge that the burdens of a continual life of pain, discomfort, immobility, dimmed consciousness, and loss of communication would not be desired by any human, and those burdens so overwhelm benefits of life that there is no obligation to assist in sustaining life. In addition, continued nutrition and hydration may have adverse consequences for the dying patient, such as the discomfort of fluid overload, aspiration, or infection at insertion sites. Also, no study has demonstrated that administered nutrition improves nutritional status or prolongs life for patients with advanced dementia, compared to patients who do not receive this intervention. Finally, it is generally agreed that deprivation of nutrients and hydration does not cause the distressing symptoms of starvation in the seriously debilitated patient, and certainly not for patients who have lost the capacity for experience, as in the vegetative state. Also, the dying patient may cease eating because of decreased metabolic requirements. Jewish scholars and Catholic theologians strongly support the moral obligation to provide nutrition for the dying. However, both admit certain specific situations in which this obligation does not hold. Jewish scholars permit refraining from artificial feeding if it causes pain and distress or in the final phases of dying. Catholic theologians have generally accepted the position that administered nutrition and hydration may be discontinued when burdens outweigh the benefits. *The Ethical and Religious Directives for Catholic Health Care Services* (2004) state: "there should be a presumption in favor of providing nutrition and hydration to all patients...as long as this is of sufficient benefit to outweigh the burdens involved to the patient." In March, 2004, Pope John Paul stated that administered nutrition and hydration were ordinary means of care and obligatory, even for patients in a vegetative state. However, in November 2004, he reaffirmed that all decisions about treatment should be based on the benefit–burden assessment of the principle of proportionality (see Section 3.3.5). At the present time, American Catholic bishops who have authority over the *Ethical and Religious Directives* are engaged in formulating a position for Catholic health care that will, in the opinion of some, take the more conservative position that artificial nutrition and hydration are always "ordinary care" and cannot be omitted.

Hamel RP, Walter JJ, eds. *Artificial Nutrition and Hydration and the Permanently Unconscious Patient. The Catholic Debate.* Washington, DC: Georgetown University Press; 2007.

In our opinion, a decision to forgo administered nutrition and hydration is ethically appropriate when: (1) no significant medical goal other than maintenance of organic life is possible; (2) the patient is so mentally incapacitated that no preferences can be expressed now or in the future; (3) no prior preferences for continued sustenance in such a situation have been expressed; and (4) the patient's situation is such that no discomfort or pain will be experienced by discontinuing the intervention. Although we acknowledge that there is some diversity of opinion on this matter, we take the position that, like all other medical interventions, the ethical propriety of nutrition and hydration should be evaluated in light of the principle of proportionality, that is, the assessment of the ratio of burdens to benefits for the patient (see Section 3.3.5).

RECOMMENDATION. In our opinion, it is ethically permissible to forgo nutrients and hydration in Mr. Care's case. He is in a vegetative state with no prognosis for recovery of consciousness and, presumably, lacks experience of any sort. He will not experience discomfort from starvation or dehydration. In Mr. B.R.'s case, opinion would be more divided. Some commentators might note that, while profoundly demented, he is still capable of experience; his continual moaning and restlessness indicate that he is uncomfortable. If discontinuing nutrients and fluids would aggravate his distress, it should not be done. However, it is unlikely that severe pain or discomfort will follow the withdrawal of nutrient support in a patient so deteriorated, and it is likely that death will occur rather quickly. Thus, it is our opinion that nutrition and hydration may be discontinued. Comfort care measures should be initiated.

Beauchamp T, Childress J. Nonmaleficence. In: Beauchamp T, Childress J, eds. *Principles of Biomedical Ethics*. 6th ed. New York, NY: Oxford University Press; 2008:113–164.

Downie R, ed. *Palliative Care Ethics: A Companion for All Specialties*. 2nd ed. New York, NY: Oxford University Press; 1999.

3.3.5 The Ethical Principle of Proportionate Treatment

The previous paragraphs have mentioned the ethical principle of proportionality. Many ethicists endorse the form of ethical reasoning that balances the intended benefits of treatment against the possible burdens. This form of reasoning is sometimes called *proportionality; namely, a medical treatment is ethically mandatory to the extent that it is likely to confer greater benefits than burdens upon the patient.* Proportionality is one way of formulating the principles of beneficence and nonmaleficence. It also includes the principle of autonomy and of satisfaction about quality of life, because the terms burdens and benefits can comprise all these ethical elements.

Proportionality is a test of the ethical obligation to recommend or provide a medical intervention: it is the estimate of its promised benefit over its attendant burdens. Although benefit–burden ratios are intrinsic to all medical decision making, it is important to notice that proportionality endorses this form of reasoning even in life–death decisions, which has often been thought to exclude such calculation in favor of an absolute duty to preserve life. In fact, some patients may view death as a benefit. Proportionality states that no absolute duty to preserve life exists; that obligation holds only when life can be judged more a benefit than a burden by and for the patient. This is a judgment ideally made by the patient but that often falls to the patient's family, surrogate, and to clinicians. Proportionality clearly applies to the patient's preferences. Patients have the right to determine what they will accept as benefits and burdens. However, proportionality also applies to medical indications. Physicians must formulate in their own minds the benefit–burden ratio to recommend appropriate options to patients or to their surrogates. Proportionality reasoning also must consider quality of life, insofar as a patient or those responsible for making decisions on the patient's behalf, view life as a benefit that is satisfactory to the patient, or a burden that the patient would reject.

We recommend that proportionality supplant other ways of formulating arguments about forgoing life support that were long used in medical ethics, such as such omission or commission, withholding or withdrawing, active or passive, and ordinary or extraordinary care. One still hears in clinical settings such remarks as, "Withholding treatment might be acceptable, but once it's started, we cannot withdraw," or "Would extubation be active or passive euthanasia?" Most ethicists consider these distinctions confusing.

Beauchamp TL, Childress JF. Distinctions and rules governing nontreatment. In: Beauchamp TL, Childress JF, eds. *Principles of Biomedical Ethics*. 6th ed. New York, NY: Oxford University Press; 2009:119–132.

President's Commission for the Study of Ethical Problems in Medicine and Biomedical and Behavioral Research. *Deciding to Forego Life-Sustaining Treatment*. Chapter 2: Elements of Good Decision making. US Government Printing Office: Washington, DC, 1983. http//:www.bioethics.gov/reports/past_commissions.

3.3.6 Legal Implications of Forgoing Life Support

The death of a patient resulting from a decision to discontinue medical intervention on the grounds of quality of life has legal implications. The cases of termination of treatment discussed in Topic One involved persons whose death was imminent and for whom further intervention was unlikely to attain medical goals. The cases in Topic Two dealt with termination of treatment that a competent patient had declined. Cases of these type are not likely to generate legal problems unless someone, such as a relative or another physician, claims the judgment of medical futility was wrongly made or that the patient's preferences were ignored. In the cases described in the present chapter, the patient could be kept alive, perhaps for some time, by continued use of the respirator, by dialysis, or by some other intervention. It is the absence of quality of that continued life that leads to the recommendation to cease intervention.

Cases where quality of life is the central issue are legally more problematic than the sort of cases described in Topics One and Two. For instance, a person who could be kept alive is allowed to die and the person's preferences are unknown. In legal theory, this might be considered homicide (although the traditional definitions of homicide certainly did not envision the problems occasioned by modern medical technology). The physician might be accused of murder or criminal negligence, or named as an accomplice in the illegal decision of another if he or she accedes to, or does not object to, the discontinuing of life support by another. A number of legal cases touching these matters have been adjudicated. We summarize some major decisions in Section 3.3.7.

It is our opinion that physicians are acting within the law, as currently understood, when they recommend that life-supporting interventions be withheld or withdrawn on grounds of quality of life, (unless specific law to the contrary exists in any particular jurisdiction) under four specific conditions: (1) It is virtually certain that further medical intervention will not attain any of the goals of medicine other than sustaining organic life; (2) the preferences of the patient are not known and cannot be expressed; (3) quality of life is severely or profoundly diminished as defined in Sections 3.3.1–3.3.3.; and (4) family are in accord. We hold this opinion because, despite the legal perplexities, most leading cases thus far adjudicated have affirmed the legal correctness of allowing the patient to die when these conditions are present. These conditions are stated in various ways in many model policies that have been prepared by local and national medical societies, specialty associations, and advocacy groups. Finally, institutions should request their legal counsels to prepare clear instructions for the medical staff in view of prevailing local law; hospital ethics committees should formulate policy that reflects these ethical conditions as well as prevailing law.

3.3.7 Judicial Decisions about Forgoing Life-Sustaining Treatment

Some important judicial decisions relevant to cases of this sort are summarized here. These summaries are brief and, given the legal complexities, are provided only to familiarize the reader with the names of the cases and the principal issues. Fuller description and the proper legal citations can be found in many places. Some resources are mentioned later.

American Medical Association. *Current Opinions with Annotations of the Ethical and Judicial Council of the American Medical Association.* Chicago, IL: AMA [issued annually].

Lo B. Legal rulings on life-sustaining interventions. In: Lo B, ed. *Resolving Ethical Dilemmas: A Guide for Clinicians.* 4th ed. Philadelphia, PA: Lippincott Williams & Wilkins; 2005:170–178.

Meisel A. *The Right to Die.* New York, NY: Wiley; 1998 [with annual supplements].

Menikoff J. *Law and Bioethics.* Washington, DC: Georgetown University Press; 2001.

The judicial decisions in this area can be divided into two categories: (1) those involving competent patients expressing a desire to have medical treatment terminated, and (2) those involving incompetent patients whose guardians wish to terminate treatment.

Competent Patients. A California appellate court determined in 1984 that the right of privacy granted by the California Constitution is broad enough to allow a competent patient to refuse all medical interventions including those that, once removed, would hasten death (*Bartling v Superior Court* 1984). The case involved a 70-year-old man suffering from multiple chronic conditions, including emphysema and a malignant tumor on his lung. The patient, who had decisional capacity, sought the removal of his ventilator; his hospital refused, concerned that the patient would die if the machine was removed. The court sided with the patient, holding that his right to have life support discontinued extends to both competent and comatose terminally ill patients.

In 1990, the United States Supreme Court stated that competent patients have a constitutionally protected interest in refusing medical treatment, extending the protections granted by the California court to the entire nation. (*Cruzan v Missouri Dept. of Health* 1990). The U.S. Supreme Court said the right was based in the term "liberty" in the 14th Amendment, whereas the California court had based the right in the California Constitution's privacy clause. Regardless of the source of the right, the end result was the same: a competent patient's protected interest in refusing medical treatment was recognized. Although the Supreme Court noted that the State's interests in preserving life, preventing suicide, and protecting the interests of third parties and the integrity of the medical profession could overrule the patient's interests, this rarely occurs in cases involving competent patients. Some legal scholars believe that the right of a competent individual to refuse life-sustaining treatment is "virtually absolute." Judicial decisions have most commonly upheld this right when patients are also suffering from terminal conditions.

Incompetent Patients. The second category of cases involves patients who are incompetent, whether caused by being comatose, mentally retarded, or otherwise impaired. In the landmark case, *In the Matter of Quinlan* (1976), the New Jersey Supreme Court held that a patient's right of privacy includes the right to refuse respiratory support that prolongs organic life when the patient is not likely to return to a "conscious and sapient condition." The plaintiffs, the parents of a young woman in a permanent vegetative state, sought a court order to remove the respirator prolonging their daughter's life. The court determined that a guardian may assert this right on behalf of a patient and that a physician's determination that the patient will not return to a "conscious and sapient condition," coupled with concurrence by a hospital ethics committee, shields the physician and the hospital from civil and criminal liability if the life support is withdrawn.

This view, which equated an incompetent patient's right to refuse treatment to that of a competent patient, endured until the mid-1980s in most jurisdictions. The decision in *Cruzan v Missouri Dept. of Health* (1990) mentioned above, further clarified the issue. The parents of Nancy Cruzan, a patient in a persistent vegetative state, petitioned the United States Supreme Court to order the removal of artificial nutrition and hydration tubes from their daughter after the Missouri Supreme Court denied their request. The U.S. Supreme Court stated that administered nutrition and hydration, like respirators, are medical interventions that can be removed at the patient's request. In the case of incompetent patients, the Court held that states may set their own standards for the strength of evidence required to prove that the incompetent patient would have forgone the treatment had she been competent. Missouri had adopted a stringent "clear and convincing evidence" standard, which has been applied by New York in similar cases (*In the Matter of O'Connor* 1988). It was not clear whether an advance directive would be required to meet this standard in Missouri, or whether an oral pronouncement of the patient's preferences would be enough, as has been held in New York (*In the Application of Eichner* 1979); there the court ruled that an incompetent patient's statements made concerning respirators while the patient was competent were sufficient evidence of the patient's preferences to permit the removal of the patient's respirator. The United States Supreme Court ordered the Missouri trial court to rehear the Cruzan case: that rehearing found that Nancy's comments to friends prior to her accident constituted the requisite clear and convincing evidence. In the case of Terri Schiavo (Florida 2003), a 41-year-old woman who had been in vegetative state for 15 years after an anoxic brain injury from a cardiac arrest, the Florida District Court authorized removal of medically administered nutrition and hydration on the testimony of Terri Schiavo's husband and legal guardian that she had told him that she would not desire life support in her situation. Some states have used lesser evidentiary standards, although the Cruzan case makes it clear that they are free to adopt the higher standard. After much litigation by the parents of Terri Schiavo, and despite the intermeddling of the Florida Governor, the United States Congress and the President, the original decision of the Florida District Court authorizing the removal of administered nutrition and hydration was upheld by all state and federal courts.

A more difficult decision is that involving an incompetent person whose preferences are unknown. These cases appear when patients have never been competent, such as individuals who have been severely retarded since birth, or when formerly competent individuals never expressed their preferences. The courts have taken two main approaches to this situation. Some courts allow the patient's guardian to make decisions for the patient, taking into account the patient's "personal value system" (*In the Matter of Jobes*, N.J. 1987). This situation presents a difficult ethical situation for guardians, who might be tempted to interject their own values into the decision-making process. Currently, all but two states accept the decisions of close relatives in similar situations, and many states will accept close friends as proxies.

Courts have also endorsed the "best interests" standard when the preferences of the patient were never known (see Section 3.0.7). This implies that death can be in the best interest of a person. The Quinlan decision clearly accepted this justification and has generally been followed. Usually, court intervention in such matters is unnecessary when physicians and family members are in agreement as to whether treatment should be withdrawn. For example, a Pennsylvania case held that a close family member of an incompetent patient may request that life support be withdrawn without a court order if two physicians diagnose the patient as being in an irreversible persistent vegetative state (*In re Fiori*, PA 1996). When family members are in conflict with each other or with physicians, attempts to mediate or negotiate the disagreement should be attempted. Such attempts may include ethics committee review, ethics consultations, psychiatric consultations, or team–family meetings. If nonjudicial efforts fail, litigation may be necessary to resolve the conflict.

3.3.8 Question Six—What are Plans and Rationale to Forgo Life-Sustaining Treatment?

If a recommendation is made by physicians to forgo life-sustaining treatment on the grounds explained earlier, and that recommendation is accepted by the patient or surrogate, plans should be made to continue care at an appropriate level. The primary goal of care now becomes relief of pain, assurance of comfort, and assisting the patient to die peacefully. Palliative care and pain relief have been discussed earlier; in care of the dying patient, however, some particular ethical questions arise.

3.4 PAIN RELIEF FOR TERMINALLY ILL PATIENTS

The quality of life of terminally ill patients is enhanced by palliative care that includes skilled application of pain-relieving drugs. Unfortunately, skilled use of pain-relieving drugs remains a rare talent in medical practice. However, palliative care medicine, based on sound research into causes and remedies of pain, is gaining acceptance as an alternative both to aggressive, futile interventions and also to the not so benign neglect of the dying patient. Competence in palliative care includes not only science and skill in managing pain but also understanding and application of ethical principles.

Undermedication is itself an ethical problem. Patients should not be kept on a drug regimen inadequate to control pain because of the ignorance of the physician or because of an ungrounded fear of addiction. Medical licensing boards in all states are extremely cautious about physicians' abuse of their authority to prescribe drugs and sometimes carry that caution to the point where their oversight inhibits appropriate medication for pain. Local medical societies, in collaboration with academic medical centers, should attempt to assist the licensing boards toward a balanced policy in this matter. Attempts to achieve adequate pain relief have another side effect, namely, the clouding of the patient's consciousness and the hindering of the patient's communication with family and friends. This consequence may be distressing to patient and family as well as ethically troubling to physicians and nurses. In such situations, sensitive attention to the patient's needs, together with skilled medical management, should lead as close as possible to the desired objective: maximum relief of pain with minimal diminution of consciousness and communication. Of course, if the patient is able to express preferences, these should be followed.

Efforts to relieve pain by opioids may entail respiratory depression, increasing risk of death (although this adverse effect is uncommon). The ethical question asks whether adequate pain relief should be compromised in order to avoid the risk of respiratory depression. Relief of pain and prolongation of life are both goals of medicine. When prolonging life is no longer a reasonable goal, relief of pain and other symptoms become the primary goal for the remainder of the patient's life. Pain medications, like most drugs, entail risks, and in the face of imminent death, a dosage regimen with higher risks, than would otherwise be tolerated, is acceptable. Certainly, pain relief should not be forgone or limited because of mere anticipation of this adverse effect. Also, the risk is greatly minimized by prescribing initial low doses of opioids and titrating up until adequate pain relief is achieved. An ethical principle, sometimes named the principle of double effect, is often used to analyze this clinical problem.

3.4.1 The Principle of Double Effect in Alleviating Pain

The principle of double effect is a form of ethical reasoning that recognizes that persons may face an unavoidable decision which will bring about inextricably linked effects, some good and desirable and the others bad and undesirable. The good effects are intended by the agent and are ethically permissible (e.g., relief of pain is a benefit); the bad effects are not intended by the agent and are ethically undesirable (e.g., depression of consciousness and risk of pulmonary infection). Proponents of this argument state that an ethically permissible effect can be allowed, even if the ethically undesirable one will inevitably follow, when the following conditions are present:

(a) The action itself is ethically good or at least neutral, that is, neither good nor bad in itself. For example, the administration of a drug is, apart from circumstances and intent, neither good nor bad.
(b) The agent must intend the good effects, not the bad effects, even though these are foreseen. For example, the physician's intention is to relieve pain, not to compromise consciousness or risk depressing respiratory function.
(c) The morally objectionable effect cannot be a means to the morally permissible one. For example, respiratory compromise is not the means to relief of pain.

In most clinical situations, these conditions are met. The intention behind administration of opioids is simply relief of pain. In some situations, however, a problem arises about condition (b): the physician and the family may wish not only to relieve pain but to hasten the dying process as well. If it can be said that the dosages administered are clinically rational, that is, no more drug is administered than is necessary for effective relief of pain, anxiety, and dyspnea, the palliative intention is primary and the action is ethical. If doses in excess of clinical necessity are given, the intention to hasten death seems primary. If this latter intention becomes primary, the action would constitute euthanasia and be judged unethical.

Beauchamp TL, Childress JF. Intended effects and merely foreseen effects. In: Beauchamp TL, Childress JF, eds. *Principles of Biomedical Ethics*. 6th ed. New York, NY: Oxford University Press; 2009:162–166.

Sulmasy D. Reinventing the rule of double effect. In: Steinbock B, ed. *The Oxford Handbook of Bioethics*. New York, NY: Oxford University Press; 2009: 144–152.

CASE I. Ms. Comfort has chronic pulmonary disease and also suffers from carcinoma of the breast with lymphangitic spread to lungs and bony metastases. She requires increasing opioid dosage for relief of pain. Her pulmonary function deteriorates so that her PO_2 is 45 and PCO_2 is 55 when she is pain free. Ms. Comfort is now receiving two tablets of 15 mg extended-release morphine every 8 hours (90 mg per 24 hours). She asks for further morphine. Her physician hesitates, fearing that further medication, given her already compromised respiratory ability, will cause Ms. Comfort's death. However, he orders 10 mg of immediate-release oral morphine every 2 hours (120 mg per 24 hours).

CASE II. A 63-year-old terminally ill woman, with widely metastatic esophageal cancer and profound malnutrition, developed peritonitis from a leaking gastrostomy tube. Attempted surgical correction of the leak was unsuccessful, and she continued to have peritonitis with severe abdominal pain. The patient and her family decide to have a morphine drip for control of pain. The dose of morphine is titrated to the patient's pain and to maintain her ability to communicate with her family. She experiences some decrease in respiratory drive and mental alertness. Six days after the morphine drip was started, the patient is no longer responsive. Her husband asks whether the inevitable could not be hastened. The attending physician dials up the morphine to 20 mg per hour. The patient lapses into coma. She dies 12 hours later.

COMMENT. The morphine drip is administered in response to pain with the knowledge that it increases the risk of respiratory depression. It should be noted that, in general, specialists in pain medication suggest that there is no absolute maximal dosage of opioids: each case must be assessed in terms of the particular patient's situation. However, it appears that in Case I, the dosage is maintained at a level needed to achieve a pain-free state. This is an appropriate application of the principle of double effect. In Case II, the dosage, at first rational, was increased to a point at which death was clearly intended. In that case, the ethical problem of whether this constitutes euthanasia is raised.

3.4.2 Palliative Sedation

The term *palliative sedation* (sometimes called *terminal sedation*) has been introduced into the discussion about care of terminally ill patients. Palliative sedation refers to the use of analgesic medications, which potentially hasten death because of their sedative side effects. This might be better described as "sedation of the imminently dying" and can be justified by the principle of double effect, as described in Section 3.4.1. As a practice, it is both common and ethical. However, the terms, and more particularly the term "terminal sedation" may be used to refer to the more controversial practice of sedating a patient to unconsciousness to relieve otherwise intractable physical symptoms, such as pain, shortness of breath, suffocation, seizures, and delirium and then withholding or withdrawing forms of life support such as ventilatory support, dialysis, administered nutrition, and hydration. The patient will die of dehydration or of respiratory or cardiac failure. No lethal dose of opioids or muscle relaxants is administered.

A dying patient may request sedation in this sense, or the patient's surrogate may do so when the patient is decisionally incapacitated. Proponents of palliative sedation consider it an ethical and legal alternative to euthanasia, as an amalgam of palliative care and forgoing of life support. Critics of this practice claim that it is unethical, because it does not observe an important provision of the principle of double effect, namely, the physician may foresee death but not intend it as a result of the action. The essential intent of the terminal sedation is to bring about death as rapidly and painlessly as possible (although it may also prolong dying).

CASE I. Mr. Care suffers from worsening debilitation of his multiple sclerosis. He is now hospitalized for treatment of a fourth recurrence of aspiration pneumonia. Although delirious from time to time, he is capable of making decisions. He is in unremitting pain from deep decubitus ulcers and constantly uncomfortable because of shortness of breath. He tells his wife and his doctor that he is exhausted, cannot tolerate the pain, and simply wants to be "put to sleep." A plan for terminal sedation is proposed to him and he accepts. A barbiturate infusion is begun. The dosage is increased until Mr. Care is deeply sedated and his pain appears to be controlled. No orders for fluids and nutrition are written.

CASE II. Mr. Care is in the late stages of multiple sclerosis. He is still living at home but is admitted to the hospital for aspiration pneumonia. His physician is confident that he will recover and return home. However, Mr. Care tells his wife and the physician that he is tired of living with his deteriorating condition. He refuses treatment for his pneumonia and refuses to eat, saying he intends to starve himself to death. He asks to be sedated in order to die comfortably.

COMMENT. In both cases, a person with decisional capacity refuses care (see Section 2.2.7). However, in Case I the patient is terminal, and the sedation is a response to intractable pain and recurring pneumonia. In Case II, the patient is not terminal and is not asking for pain relief but for death to be hastened. In the first case, palliative sedation is an acceptable example of double effect reasoning; in the second, palliative sedation, although not the cause of death, accelerates it. This is not ethically acceptable.

Palliative sedation in the setting of competent request and imminent death is clearly ethical. In other cases, it is ethically problematic. As a clinical practice, it should be approached cautiously. It has potential for abuse. It can become a means of enabling death of the nonterminally ill, as in Case II, or a routine clinical practice for patients who are terminal and whose wishes are not known.

3.5 MEDICALLY ASSISTED DYING

Some persons may conclude that the quality of their life is so diminished that life is no longer worth living. This conclusion may be the result of unrelieved pain or suffering, or because they consider the prospect of deterioration, or because they believe that their lives are a burden on others. Persons who come to this conclusion are often terminally ill and under the care of a physician. It may occur to them to ask their physician to help them die quickly and painlessly. In the previous sections of this book, we have discussed situations in which some form of medical treatment, such as dialysis, mechanical ventilation, or chemotherapy, was sustaining the life of the patient. We have analyzed the situations in which patients and physicians may decide to forgo these forms of medical intervention. In this section, we envision a situation in which termination of treatment will not itself cause the death of the patient; some additional action must be taken to do so. We here ask what physicians may ethically do to respond to patients' request to help them end their lives.

3.5.1 Euthanasia

The term *euthanasia*, meaning "a good death" has been used for centuries to describe this moral question. In its original medical use, "euthanasia" implied the duty of a doctor to assure that his patients died as peacefully and comfortably as the medicine of the time could provide. Direct killing was repudiated. Later, the term was used as a synonym for *mercy killing*, that is, deliberately and directly killing a sufferer to relieve pain, either by a physician or by some other compassionate party. Then, distinctions were made between voluntary, nonvoluntary, and involuntary euthanasia. Voluntary euthanasia described situations in which the patient consciously and deliberately requested death. Nonvoluntary euthanasia described situations in which the patient was decisionally incapacitated and made no request. Involuntary euthanasia described situations in which the patients were killed against their wishes. Involuntary euthanasia (practiced as a policy in Nazi medicine) has been condemned by all commentators. Nonvoluntary euthanasia, that is, causing death, usually of persons without decisional capacity, without their expressed wish, has been criticized by most commentators. Voluntary euthanasia, though very controversial, has been defended by a few commentators as ethically permissible on the basis of patient autonomy.

The contemporary debate in the United States has moved away from these distinctions and now focuses on the more precise question of whether physicians may respond to a request from a competent and terminally ill patient for assistance in dying. This question itself requires clarification. It may refer either to a situation in which a patient requests a physician to administer a lethal drug, or to a situation in which the patient asks a physician to prescribe potentially lethal medications that the patient can self-administer to bring about death. The patient makes the final decision about whether his or her quality of life is too low to continue to live. This patient performs the action that will end his or her life. By comparing this issue to the discussion about forgoing life support, it is possible to clarify similarities and differences.

EXAMPLE. Ms. Comfort is dying from widely disseminated cancer and is suffering intense pain, even though she is receiving high doses of morphine. She is conscious and capable of communication. She begs her doctor "to put her to sleep forever." The physician administers a lethal dose of a short-acting barbiturate and morphine sulfate intravenously.

COMMENT. This is an example of voluntary euthanasia: the patient requests death and the physician administers a lethal drug. The debate over the physician's role was long posed in these terms. It is obvious, in this case, that the physician is the agent and cause of the death of the patient, even though the patient voluntarily requested him to do so. However, in American law, this scenario would constitute an illegal taking of human life. In all ethics statements of medical organizations, it is considered unethical behavior. In the bioethical literature, it remains highly debatable. Today, the discussion of physician involvement in aiding the death of a patient has shifted to the formulation commonly called "physician-assisted dying," as explained later.

Beauchamp TL, Childress JF. The justification of intentionally arranged death. In: Beauchamp TL, Childress JF, eds. *Principles of Biomedical Ethics*. 6th ed. New York, NY: Oxford University Press; 2009:176–186.

Dickens BM, Boyle JM, Ganzini L. Euthansia and assisted suicide. In: Singer PA, ed. *The Cambridge Textbook of Biomedical Ethics*. New York, NY: Cambridge University Press; 2008:72–78.

Dworkin G. Physician assisted death: the state of the debate. In: Steinbock B, ed. *The Oxford Handbook of Bioethics*. New York, NY: Oxford University Press; 2009:375–393.

Lo B. Physician-assisted suicide and active euthanasia. In: Lo B, ed. *Resolving Ethical Dilemmas: A Guide for Clinicians*. 4th ed. Philadelphia, PA: Lippincott Williams & Wilkins; 2009:151–161.

3.5.2 Physician-Assisted Dying

In traditional discussions of euthanasia, the physician's role was generally described as administration of a lethal drug, usually by injection. In the more recent debates, the physician's role has been more precisely defined as the legalization of the physician's prescription of a drug that the patient may take to bring about death.

EXAMPLE. Ms. Comfort is dying from widely disseminated cancer and is suffering intense and implacable pain because of bone metastases, even with optimum pain management. She requests her physician to prescribe a supply of barbiturates sufficient for her to end her life, to give her instructions about appropriate dosage and administration, and to be present when she takes the prescribed medication to end her life.

COMMENT.

(a) Proponents of physician-assisted dying offer the following argument in its favor. It is correct, they say, that direct administration of a lethal drug constitutes an act of homicide. However, prescription of drugs that the terminally ill patient can take at will removes the physician as the agent of the patient's death. The decision and the action of ending life remain in the patient's control. The patient, then, hastens his or her own dying process, which is quite different from a suicide by a person who is not terminally ill (see Section 3.6.1). These advocates propose that the physician's participation by providing the means should be explicitly exempted from statutes that prohibit aiding a suicide. Physician participation, they claim, is a proper medical response of respect for patient autonomy and of their patient's evaluation of their quality of life.

(b) Physicians opposed to assisting patients in hastening their death in this manner regard participation as unprofessional and unethical. The American Medical Association rejects physician-assisted dying as "fundamentally incompatible with the physician's role as healer." The American College of Physicians does not support the legalization of physician-assisted dying because "the practice might undermine patient trust and distract from reform in end-of-life care" and because of the risk of discrimination against vulnerable populations, including the elderly and the disabled.

AMA Council on Ethical and Judicial Affairs, *Curr Opin.* 1996;2:211.
American College of Physicians. *American College of Physicians Ethics Manual.* 5th ed. Philadelphia, PA: American College of Physicians; 2005.

(c) The states of Oregon and of Washington are the only American jurisdictions that allow physician-assisted dying. Their statutes state that physicians may prescribe, but not administer, a lethal drug for a competently requesting patient who is terminally ill. A 2-week waiting period between request and prescription is required. The physician must be confident that the patient is making a competent and informed request, and psychiatric consultation is required if the physician suspects that the requesting patient suffers from mental illness. It is the patient rather than the physician who is in control of the process, from its initiation to its completion. This feature of assisted dying differentiates it ethically and legally from other legalized forms of euthanasia, such as in the Netherlands and Belgium, where physicians are permitted to be the agents of the patient's death.

Since 1997, when physician-assisted suicide was legalized in Oregon, approximately 0.1% of Oregon deaths (about 30–60 out of approximately 38,000 annually) have resulted from physician-assisted dying. Also, some patients who obtain a prescription never make use of it. Only a small number of physicians and patients participate in physician-assisted dying. Any physician may decline to participate. The reasons most commonly offered for requests are controlling the timing of death, not becoming dependent, and avoiding future pain (rather than actual pain in the present).

3.5.3 Ethical Arguments

The public, the medical community, and medical ethicists are divided about the ethical propriety of physician-assisted dying. The opponents offer the following arguments:

(a) Prohibition of direct taking of human life has been a central tenet of many religious traditions and has been equally strong in the secular ethic. An ancient maxim of the Western legal tradition states that even the consent of the victim is not a defense against homicide. These opponents consider the "indirect" involvement of the physician as only a prescriber, not an administrator, of the lethal intervention as equally objectionable.

(b) Medical ethics has traditionally emphasized the saving and preservation of life and has repudiated the direct taking of life. The Hippocratic Oath states: "I will not administer a deadly poison to anyone when asked to do so nor suggest such a course." This ancient prohibition seems directly aimed at physician-assisted dying. Contemporary organized medicine reaffirms this tradition.

(c) The dedication of the medical profession to the welfare of patients and to the promotion of health might be seriously undermined in the eyes of the public and of patients by the participation of physicians in the death of the very ill, even of those who request it.

(d) Requests for swift death are often made in circumstances of extreme distress, which may be alleviated by skillful pain management and other positive interventions such as those employed in hospice care. Similarly, such requests may manifest a treatable depression.

(e) Even if approval is limited to voluntary assisted dying, it is possible that, once established, the practice might become tolerated for nonvoluntary patients whom others assume "would have requested it" if they had been able. Similarly, the availability of quick death may bring subtle coercion on persons who feel that their compromised state is a burden to others. Therefore, even when effecting a swift death at the request of a suffering patient seems merciful and benevolent, the acceptance of the practice as ethical may bear the seeds of dangerous social consequences. This is the so-called slippery-slope argument, namely, that tolerance for a practice on the grounds that it is harmless in one situation will gradually lead to tolerance of similar but more dangerous practices. In the Netherlands, where euthanasia is legal, some commentators claim there is such a slide; no similar slide has appeared in the state of Oregon.

Proponents of physician-assisted dying counter with the following arguments:

(a) The termination of treatment in many cases hastens a patient's death, such as discontinuing artifical nutrition and hydration for a patient in a vegetative state, who is not even terminally ill. Permitting competent and conscious but terminally ill patients to decide to hasten their death is less ethically problematic.

(b) Autonomous individuals have moral authority over their lives; patients who are dying should be allowed the means to control the time and manner of their death with assistance from competent clinicians.

(c) No person should be required to bear disproportionate burdens of pain and suffering, and those who relieve them of such burdens, at their request, are acting ethically, that is, out of compassion and respect for autonomy. Physicians do not have a duty to prescribe lethal drugs; they are ethically permitted to accept or reject the terminally ill patient's request.

(d) Often the burdens of pain and disability are the result of the "success" of medical intervention that has extended life of unacceptable quality. Those who have effected this result should be permitted to respect the patient's desire no longer to bear so unrewarding a result. Just as patients may refuse artificial nutrition and hydration to hasten their death, one might argue that physician-assisted dying accomplishes the same goal.

(e) The maxim of the Hippocratic Oath prohibiting the "giving of poisons" is outdated, because medicine could never have anticipated the ability to prolong dying that it has today.

(f) Some voices within the medical profession, which has been tradition-ally opposed to euthanasia, have recently expressed support for the carefully circumscribed forms of assistance in dying that have been legalized in Oregon and Washington State.

COMMENT. These arguments are vigorously debated by proponents and op-ponents of physician-assisted dying. During the 1990s, efforts were made, by legislation and by judicial decision, to make physician-assisted dy-ing legal. Oregon and Washington states have done so. The United States Supreme Court has ruled that, while there is no constitutional right to physician-assisted dying, states may legislate either to prohibit or to permit it (*Washington v Glucksberg* and *Vacco v Quill* 1997).

3.5.4 Physician Response to Request for Assistance in Dying

Even though physician-assisted dying may be widely legalized in the fu-ture, debates about its ethical propriety will continue. Physicians will have to make conscientious decisions about whether to provide assistance to patients to hasten their deaths. The practice of physician-assisted dying requires difficult decisions about what constitutes terminal illness, and whether all means of relieving physical and psychological pain have been exhausted. In particular, legal authorization limited to only competent pa-tients in terminal illness leaves unanswered questions about patients in equally distressing circumstances who are unable to self-administer lethal medication and also about persons who are not terminal but who anticipate slow death from degenerative disease. In addition, the question of how vigorously to pursue diagnosis of mental illness, especially depression, remains unsettled.

A request from a patient for assistance in dying should be met in the following manner:

(a) A physician who is unpersuaded by the arguments supporting physician-assisted dying must inform the patient that he or she can-not in conscience cooperate. This physician should offer to discuss the issue in depth with the patient, in hope of finding mutually acceptable options. If the patient continues to request assistance, the physician may offer to resign from the case or to provide only palliative care.

(b) A physician who is persuaded by the arguments favoring assisted dying must recognize that assisting is illegal except in Oregon and Washington. Different jurisdictions have somewhat differing laws and different ways of dealing with the issue, but, in general, assisting a patient to die by prescribing a lethal drug is a criminal act. A physician may choose to take the risk of legal liability, but should do so in full knowledge of the possible consequences.

(c) If a physician chooses to take the legal risk, he or she should be confident that the patient has decisional capacity and is suffering from a condition that can realistically be characterized as terminal. Consultation on these matters is advisable.

(d) The physician should explore the issue with the patient very carefully and sympathetically. The patient's medical situation, options for treatment, alternatives ways to hasten death, palliative care, relief of pain, social supports, values, and attitudes should be discussed. The discussion should take place over time and might include others, such as the patient's spouse and children, closest friends, and religious and ethical counselors.

3.6 CARE OF THE DYING PATIENT

Quality end-of-life care requires a combination of the judgment of clinicians and the preferences of patients in three particular areas, namely, achieving appropriate control of pain and symptoms, avoiding inappropriate prolongation of dying, and enhancing the control of patients over their care. Other aspects of quality care rest primarily with patient and family, supported by physicians, nurses, and social workers. Spiritual concerns of the patient should be met in ways congenial to the patient.

A decision to terminate some specific form of treatment or not to resuscitate does not imply the termination of other forms of care for the patient. It is frequently noted that after a DNR order is written, attention to the patient's needs diminishes. This is unethical for two reasons. First, more than 50% of patients for whom DNR orders have been written survive to be discharged. These patients require continued appropriate care. Second, when the goals of curing are exhausted, the goals of caring must be reinforced. In hospice care, life-support technology and life-saving interventions are avoided in favor of comfort care. Attention to relief of pain and discomfort and enhancement of the patient's ability to interact with family and friends become predominant goals. Hospice care and palliative medicine work to achieve these goals. The medical proverb is pertinent: cure sometimes, provide relief as often as possible, comfort always.

3.7 TREATMENT OF ATTEMPTED OR SUSPECTED SUICIDES

Suicide is the deliberate taking of one's life. It is natural to assume that attempted suicide in part reflects a personal belief that the quality of one's life has become unbearable because of mental illness, significant personal losses, overwhelming emotional conflicts, or impulsive decisions.

3.7.1 Question Seven—What is the Legal and Ethical Status of Suicide?

If a person has made a life-threatening suicide attempt (or suspected suicide attempt) and is brought to an emergency room, the patient should be stabilized in accordance with the Emergency Medical Treatment and Labor Act. Even when a suicide attempt is supported by evidence, such as a history and a suicide note, it is customary to provide all means necessary for resuscitation and care on the presumption that the suicide attempt is a result of mental illness.

CASE. Ms. D.W., a 24-year-old woman, is brought to the ED; she has overdosed and deeply slashed her wrists. She is obtunded. She has been brought in several times before and is known to have a psychiatric history of depression. On her last admission, she screamed that next time she should be allowed to die.

RECOMMENDATION. Ms. D.W. should be treated. The customary practice of disregarding the suicide wish in the emergency department situation is ethically appropriate. The following comments are pertinent to this situation:

(a) The ethical basis for suicide prevention is the well-authenticated psychological thesis that the suicide attempt is often a "cry for help" rather than an unambivalent decision to end one's life. Frequently, the fact that the attempted suicide arrives in the ED suggests the act was ambivalently motivated. Many suicide attempts are halfway. The suicide attempt may not be an act of autonomy but rather be an act resulting from impaired capacity because of a mental or physical disease or emotional conflict.

(b) Suicide attempts are often undertaken in psychopathological conditions, such as depression, that are treatable or under social conditions that are transient, such as disappointed love or financial loss. It is sometimes possible to anticipate these problems. Physicians have an ethical obligation to recognize the suicidal inclinations of patients whom they encounter in their practice and to make efforts to assist them personally or by referral to a trained suicide counselor or a psychiatrist.

3.7.2 Suicide and Refusal of Treatment

It is sometimes asked whether refusal of treatment by a patient, especially a patient who is terminally ill, is equivalent to suicide. If it were, the physician might feel constrained to prevent suicide or to avoid complicity. Significant ethical differences exist between suicide and refusal of medical care. Following are examples of these differences:

(a) In refusal of care, persons do not take their lives; instead they do not permit another to help them survive. Persons who abhor the thought of suicide may say, "I do not want to kill myself. I only want to be allowed to die on my own terms and to control the time and manner of my dying."

(b) In refusal of care, death is caused by the progress of a lethal disease, which is not treated; in suicide, the immediate cause of death is a self-inflicted lethal act. In refusing life-saving care, the patient does not set in motion the lethal cause. The patient's refusal authorizes the physician to refrain from therapy; the fatal condition is itself the cause of death.

(c) Even though suicide and refusal of treatment both result in death, the moral setting differs completely in intention, circumstances, motives, and desires.

(d) The Roman Catholic Church condemns suicide. It does permit its adherents to refuse care, even should death result, when treatment is "extraordinary," that is, offers little hope and is excessively burdensome, painful, or costly.

(e) Many judicial decisions and legal statutes now distinguish between legitimate refusal of care and suicide. Most Advance Directive legislation explicitly states that death following a decision authorized by these acts cannot be considered suicide for purposes of denial of life insurance.

3.7.3 Legal Status of Suicide

Suicide was once a criminal act in the Anglo-American common law, but all sanctions for suicide (which formerly had included confiscation of the suicide's estate) were repealed in American jurisdictions in the nineteenth century. Although suicide is not illegal, state laws do support suicide prevention. In all states, involuntary psychiatric treatment may be given to persons considered "a danger to themselves" by possible suicide. Also, most jurisdictions retain legal sanctions against aiding and abetting suicides. These laws apply to anyone who, under current law, provides physician-assisted dying for terminally ill patients except in the states of Oregon and Washington.

3P PEDIATRIC NOTES

3.1P Features of Quality-of-Life Judgments for Infants and Children

Quality-of-life judgments about children differ from those made about adults in two important ways. First, adults often can express preferences about future states of life and health. Second, when an adult is incapable of expressing preferences, the history of that person's preferences and style of life often allows others to estimate how that person would value and adapt to future situations. In pediatrics, the life whose quality is being assessed is almost entirely in the future. Also, just as in adult care, pediatricians tend to assess quality of life as lower than either parents or the affected children.

Medical interventions that are generally effective in alleviating physical disability are ethically mandatory when the only supposed contraindication is developmental disabilities in the range characteristic of Down syndrome. More complicated medical conditions, such as major cardiac deformity, may be genuine contraindications to treatment.

3.2P Best Interest Standard for Children

Children have little or no history of preferences on which to base a surrogate judgment. The first standard for surrogate decisions, substituted judgment, is not relevant. All surrogate judgments for minor children must adhere to the best interest standard (see Section 3.0.7).

In some particularly difficult cases, the ethical question is whether the quality of future life for each of these children justifies a decision to proceed or refrain from medical interventions that will sustain life. Parents and physicians will reach their conclusions based on many factors. We note here several factors that are, in our opinion, of importance. First, one major factor is whether or not these cases represent what some have called *qualitative futility*, that is, some goal may be successfully attained but that goal is not worth achieving. In other terms, the experiences of the person would be considered undesirable by the one living it and by most objective observers. In Section 3.3.1, we distinguish diminished quality of life into restricted, severely diminished, and profoundly diminished. Second, the prognoses that such quality of life will eventuate is often quite different. The degree of certitude attached to any clinical judgment is controversial, but some judgments rest on better and more extensive experience and data than others.

Determining the course of action that is in the child's best interests is not always easy. Parents have a fundamental right to direct the upbringing of their children in such a way so as to be consistent with their values, and this right is generally thought to extend to medical decision making. In determining the course of action that is in the child's best interests, the expected benefits of a treatment must be balanced against a parent's right to control the child's medical care in accordance with the family's values and beliefs.

Frankel LR, Goldworth A, Rorty MV, Silverman WA. *Ethical Dilemmas in Pediatrics*. Part II. Medical Futility. New York, NY: Cambridge University Press; 2005:89–157.

Contextual Features

This broadly titled topic is essential to the description and resolution of a case in clinical ethics. It addresses the ways in which professional, familial, religious, financial, legal, and institutional factors influence clinical decisions. These factors are the context in which the case occurs and so we call this topic *Contextual Features*. Although clinical ethics focuses on medical indications, patient preferences, and quality of life in particular cases of patient care, medical decisions are not simply individual choices by two autonomous agents (the physician and the patient). Choices are influenced and constrained by contextual considerations.

Today, the encounter between patient and physician occurs in more complex institutional and economic structures than ever before. Only occasionally does the traditional private relationship exist in which a patient chooses and consults a physician in private practice and pays a fee out of pocket for service. More often, doctors have multiple relationships with other physicians, nurses, allied health professionals, health care administrators, insurers, professional organizations, and state and federal agencies, in addition to their own families. Similarly, the relationship between a patient and a physician is surrounded by the patient's family and friends, other health professionals, and the hospital as an institution. The complex relationships between medicine and the pharmaceutical industry burden patients and create conflicts of interest for physicians. Physicians and patients are also subject to the varying influence of community and professional standards, legal rules, governmental and institutional policies about financing and access to health care, computerized methods of storage and retrieval of medical information, the relationship between research and practice, and other factors.

Physicians often perceive these contextual features as conflicting with their primary commitment to individual patients—and they often do. Some physicians might believe that contextual factors are, or should be, of little or no relevance in an ethical decision about patient care: his or her duties

161

are narrowly focused on the patient. We consider this view obsolete and theoretically incorrect. Many of the factors mentioned previously impose responsibilities and duties on both patients and physicians. The ethical task is to determine how correctly to assess the importance of these contextual features in a particular case.

These contextual features can be viewed from the large perspective of social policy. Indeed, the serious discussions about reform of the health care system takes place at this level. Many bioethicists address questions of health policy, which are subjected to ethical analysis under the rubric of justice. Certainly, the currently distorted organization of American health care does contribute to ethical complexities that arise in patient care, and, often, these complexities cannot be resolved apart from institutional reform. Still, the focus of this book is on clinical cases that arise and must be managed medically and ethically within extant structures. Those who desire to learn more about the ethics of health policy may consult the large bioethical literature on justice and health care.

Daniels N, Sabin J. *Setting Limits Fairly: Can We Learn to Share Medical Resources?* New York, NY: Oxford University Press; 2002.

Danis M, Clancy C, Churchill L. *Ethical Dimensions of Health Policy.* New York, NY: Oxford University Press; 2002.

Rhodes R, Battin HP, Silver A. *Medicine and Social Justice. Essays on the Distribution of Health Care.* New York, NY: Oxford University Press; 2002.

4.0.1 Ethical Principles in Contextual Features

It is difficult to designate a single ethical principle that might be relevant to all contextual features. In all of the questions examined in Topic Four, we are faced with decisions that confront doctors and patients because they encounter each other within the complex and often misshapen structures of health care, and within social and cultural institutions over which they have little control.

The principles we have seen in other topic areas, namely, beneficence and respect for autonomy intersect with contextual features. However, bioethicists commonly add the ethical principle of justice to their list of significant principles. *Justice refers to those moral and social theories that attempt to distribute the benefits and burdens of a social system in a fair and equitable way among all participants in the system.* This conception of justice is highly relevant to health policy and health care reform. For the contextual problems in clinical ethics, we select a narrower part of this broad idea of justice, namely, fairness. Fairness is a moral characteristic relevant to transactions and relationships between individuals. In games, fairness requires "playing by the rules"; in business, fairness requires "a level playing field." *In general, fairness demands that transactions and relationships give to each participant that which they deserve and reasonably expect. In addition, it is obviously unfair to exploit by deceit, manipulation, or discrimination.*

Beauchamp TL, Childress JF. Justice. In: Beauchamp TL, Childress JF, eds. *Principles of Biomedical Ethics*. 6th ed. New York, NY: Oxford University Press, 2009:240–280.

4.0.2 Conflict of Interest

The context in which a therapeutic relationship takes place can often give rise to conflicts of interest. Indeed, the therapeutic relationship itself involves a potential conflict of interest: the physician has knowledge and skill needed by a vulnerable person, the patient, and has the power to benefit personally by exploiting that vulnerability. However, the basic ethics of the therapeutic relationship, beneficence and respect for autonomy are intended to preserve that relationship from exploitation. When we view the relationship within the larger picture of contextual features, we see conflicts of interest that must be eliminated or managed in ways that do not damage the relationship. Thus, in this chapter, conflict of interest appears as a consistent theme.

The term conflict of interest is often used to describe a situation in which a person might be motivated to perform actions that his or her professional role makes possible but that are at variance with the acknowledged duties of that role. The term was first applied to political office holders and judges whose power to dispense money, power, or punishment might be enticed away from the public good or the law by the lure of personal profit. More recently, the concept has been applied to other professions, including medicine.

A potential conflict of interest is not in itself unethical. When an individual is provided the opportunity to gain personal benefit by acting contrary to duty, he or she may never take advantage of that opportunity, despite incentives that may be difficult to resist. If a potential conflict of interest does not result in unfair treatment, no ethical violation has occurred. It should be noted that, while we treat conflict of interest as a matter of fairness, violations that arise from conflicts of interest can also be seen as doing harm (maleficence) and as unprofessional behavior deserving of sanctions.

Fairness demands that those values most associated with the professional duty of the decision maker should rank highly in resolving the conflict. Judges are publically expected to make equitable decisions based on the facts and the law; plaintiffs and defendants have the right to a fair hearing. Similarly, physicians should honor their professional commitment to the welfare of their patients; patients have a right to honest diagnosis and indicated treatment, as well as to be treated with respect. Commitment to fairness in relationships is the primary means to control conflicts of interest. However, in situations where conflicts of interest may be pervasive and powerful, certain public measures such as disclosure, recusal from the case, or legal prohibitions with sanctions, may be useful and necessary.

4.0.3 Contents of This Topic

Under the topic of contextual features, we discuss: (1) professional conflicts of interest that might affect clinical decisions; (2) the role of interested parties other than the patient, such as the patient's family; (3) confidentiality of medical information; (4) financial arrangements that might insert conflicts of interest into clinical decisions; (5) allocation of scarce health resources; (6) the role of religion; (6) the role of the law; (7) clinical research and teaching; (8) medical research and medical teaching; (9) public health; and (10) organizational ethics, specifically the roles of ethics committees and ethics consultation within the health care institution.

We ask 10 questions about Contextual Features that are relevant to the analysis of an ethical problem.

1. Are there professional, interprofessional, or business interests that might create conflicts of interest in the clinical treatment of patients?
2. Are there parties other than clinicians and patients, such as family members, who have an interest in clinical decisions?
3. What are the limits imposed on patient confidentiality by the legitimate interests of third parties?
4. Are there financial factors that create conflicts of interest in clinical decisions?
5. Are there problems of allocation of scarce health resources that might affect clinical decisions?
6. Are there religious issues that might influence clinical decisions?
7. What are the legal issues that might affect clinical decisions?

8. Are there considerations of clinical research and education that might affect clinical decisions?
9. Are there issues of public health and safety that affect clinical decisions?
10. Are there conflicts of interest within institutions and organizations (e.g., hospitals) that may affect clinical decisions and patient welfare?

4.1 HEALTH PROFESSIONS

4.1.1 Question One—Are There Professional, Interprofessional, or Business Interests That Might Create Conflicts of Interest in the Clinical Treatment of Patients?

A profession is an occupation requiring special learning or science, together with competency utilized in the service of others. Its members profess commitment to competence, integrity, and dedication to the good of their clients and the public. In return, society grants professions a wide scope of self-regulation in admission of members, their education, their discipline and forms of practice. The health professions state their commitments in oaths and codes of ethics. A renewed interest in professionalism has led major medical organizations to formulate *The Physician's Charter*. This document states three fundamental principles of professionalism: the principle of primacy of patient welfare, the principle of patient autonomy, and the principle of social justice. The principle of patient welfare and of patient autonomy are treated in Topic One and Topic Two of this book. This Topic "Contextual Features" discusses the way in which the *primacy* of the principle of patient welfare, which requires loyalty between patient and physician can be realized within the constraints of broad social arrangements of health care.

4.1.2 The Multiple Responsibilities of Physicians

The ethics of medicine has traditionally directed the physician to attend primarily to the needs of the patient. It is clearly unethical for a physician to do anything to a patient that is not intended to benefit the patient but rather only to benefit the physician or some other party. For example, a physician who performs diagnostic or therapeutic procedures that are not indicated, under pretense of caring for the patient but with the intent only of collecting a fee, clearly acts unethically. In recent years, the absorption of the once very private relationship between physicians and patients into large organizations that employ or contract with physicians and that enroll and insure patients has added a new dimension to the physician's duties. These dimensions may not be unethical but may create conflicts of interest that may be unethical. Frequently, physicians take on contractual obligations with these organizations that directly affect the ways in which they care for their patients. Similarly, many opportunities to profit from professional identity and knowledge are presented by association with pharmaceutical companies and by investment in organizations that provide clinical services. Another ethical problem is posed when multiple responsibilities make it difficult to determine which responsibilities have priority in a particular case, such as when the duty to one's patient is in conflict with duties to others. We discuss this issue in Section 4.5.

Medical professionalism in the new millennium: a physician charter. *Ann Intern Med.* 2002;136:244–246.
Medical professionalism in the new millennium: a physician charter. *Lancet.* 2002;359:520–522.

4.1.3 Allegiance and Altruism

The Physician's Charter states, "The principle of the primacy of patient welfare is based on a dedication to serving the interest of the patient. Altruism contributes to the trust that is central to the physician–patient relationship. Market forces, societal pressures, and administrative exigencies must not compromise this principle." The Merriman Webster dictionary defines "altruism" as "unselfish concern for the welfare of others; selflessness." The term "altruism" is a rather exaggerated expression of the nature of a professional relationship. It implies that a physician must always act out of selfless motives and that duties toward patients always supercede other obligations and responsibilities. We prefer to use the term *allegiance, that is, a particularly compelling, though not exclusive, commitment to a cause, a community, or person.* All persons have multiple allegiances or loyalties—to family, to friends, to a religious faith, to a community, to a nation, to a cause—and usually these can be managed without conflict. At times, different loyalties will pull a person in opposite directions, and then a choice must be made. Also, there are allegiances that are immoral, such as to a violent cause. The tradition of medical ethics, the expectations of the public, and the common law assign a high priority to the physician's allegiance to his or her patients. Still, other allegiances and moral duties may put constraints on the physician's allegiance to individual patients. When policies are fairly and justly developed for the distribution of some good, such as transplantable organs or medicines in epidemics, individual physicians are obliged to adhere to these rules even if such adherence compromises each patient's interests.

Beauchamp TL, Childress JF. Patient-physician relationships. In: Beauchamp TL, Childress JF, eds. *Principles of Biomedical Ethics.* 6th ed. New York, NY: Oxford University Press; 2009:288–332.
Lo B. Overview of the Doctor-patient relationship. In: Lo B, ed. *Resolving Ethical Dilemmas.* 3rd ed. Philadelphia, PA: Lippincott Williams and Wilkins; 2005:155–156.

4.1.4 Cooperation Between Medical and Nursing Professionals

Physicians interact with other professionals, in particular with nurses. Nursing is a profession that has its own ethical traditions and standards, which stress a strong loyalty toward their patients. Ideally, the relationship between physicians and nurses is cooperative and collaborative. However, on occasion, nurses may believe that a patient is not being well served by the attending physicians. This can often be clarified by respectful conversation. Yet, the difference in status between physicians and nurses can inhibit this sort of solution. In such situations, ethicists speak of "moral distress . . . when one knows the right thing to do but institutional constraints make it nearly impossible to pursue the right course of action" (Jameton). Many studies show that moral distress is common in the clincial setting where nurses feel constrained by the hierarchy of power relationships or by administrative structures. These studies show that the presence of moral distress negatively affects the care of patient. Although moral distress has been most fully explored in nursing, it also applies to other interprofessional relations involving differences in status, such as between medical students, house officers, and attendings. It is imperative to recognize this problem and to take interpersonal and institutional steps to remedy it. One approach that is often helpful is the use of ethics consultation and ethics committee deliberation, which can reduce the adverse effects of hierarchical relations among professionals.

Jameton A. *Nursing Practice: The Ethical Issues.* New York, NY: Prentice-Hall; 1984.

4.1.5 Relations Between Physicians and Medically Related Business

The relationships that physicians may have with medically related businesses are rife with conflicts of interest. Physicians may interact with businesses in many ways. Their relationship with their hospitals, their financial investments in health care activities, their contacts with pharmaceutical industry may influence clinical decisions.

EXAMPLE I. Physicians in a small city are regularly invited to lunches and dinners at fine restaurants by a pharmaceutical firm. The gatherings are billed as "Gourmet Knowledge," and feature a distinguished speaker addressing issues in health care and treatment. The sponsor's products are mentioned but only together with competing products in a "scientific and impartial commentary."

EXAMPLE II. A group of internists in a small, semi-rural city, intend to invest in a clinical laboratory to which they can refer their patients, instead of sending them for tests to the local hospital laboratories.

EXAMPLE III. A university general medicine practice provides cares for many patients who are capitated under federal and state programs. The practice recruits physicians by financially rewarding the practice of evidence-based medicine. The practice offers a generous incentive program, with bonuses up to 30% of base salary, if physicians avoid high-cost interventions that have not been established as cost-effective in caring for a group of capitated patients.

COMMENT. Each of these cases presents a conflict of interest. Some conflicts of interest can be eliminated by law. The physicians in Example II know that federal legislation prohibits physicians from making referrals of a Medicare or Medicaid patient to an entity that furnishes designated health services (including laboratory services) in which the physician has a financial interest. This law (Stark Law, 1989, 1993, 1994) virtually outlaws self-referral. However, the Stark law is extremely complex and does allow a variety of exceptions. In this case, the physicians seek legal advice whether they can use two of these exemptions, namely, the ancillary services and the rural practitoner provisions. Other conflicts can be discouraged. For example, a hospital may discourage drug representatives from providing food for meetings, but does not sanction that behavior, leaving implementation to individual departments. One of the most common ways of dealing with conflicts of interest is to require that they be clearly disclosed to the parties involved as well as appropriately managed. If a party involved in a conflict of interest discloses it, the second party can take some protective action, such as leaving the relationship or guarding against some action contrary to his or her interests. In professional relationships, where one party, the professional person, often possesses the advantage of special knowledge, this disclosure may not be effective. It may be necessary for the professional to recuse himself or herself from the relationship or discard the conflicting aspects of it.

RECOMMENDATION. In Example I, Gourmet Knowledge provides a subtle but highly effective influence on physicians to view favorably the products of the sponsor. Many studies demonstrate that, despite physicians' honest belief that they are not influenced, they are swayed by such attention. Example II, the prospect of profit to the physician–owners of the laboratory may influence their clinical judgments about the need for diagnostic testing for their patients. Because their plan clearly raises the application of the Stark laws, they may attempt to avoid it by manipulation of the terms of the exceptions. If they succeed in so doing, they constitute themselves in a moral, if not legal, conflict of interest. They must scrupulously abide by the regulations governing the exceptions. They should declare their ownership to patients for whom they prescribe testing. They should follow the advice of the American Medical Association's Council on Ethics and Legal Affairs. This statement asks whether some social need justifies establishment of such an entity. This places a heavy ethical burden on the conscience of the physicians. They may ignore it and run the risk of being branded as unethical, or they may seriously take the problem of exploiting patients and establish some sort of impartial record review to assure appropriateness of referrals. In Case III, the organization that devised the incentive program has an obligation to design the program in a way that assures the freedom of clinicians to order appropriate care. The program should be explained to patients as a means of effective and efficient care that does not limit or ration appropriate treatment.

Brennan TA et al. Health industry practices that create conflicts of interest: a policy proposal for academic medical centers. *JAMA.* 2006;295:429–433.

4.1.6 Physician's Duty to Self and Family

Another area of potential conflict concerns the physician's need to attend to his or her personal well-being and to that of their family. Every physician, like every human being, has certain moral duties to self, to spouse and children, and to colleagues. Every health professional must find the balances and compromises that reconcile duties to patients with these personal and familial responsibilties. Failure to mangage these relationships leads to personal distress, decline in health, family crises, and diminished ability to care for patients. In recent years, many professional organizations have established programs to educate and support professionals who find themselves torn between these duties.

4.2 OTHER INTERESTED PARTIES

4.2.1 Question Two—Are There Parties Other Than Clinicians and Patients, Such as Family Members, Who Have an Interest in Clinical Decisions?

The primary interested parties in a clinical relationship are the patient and the physician, along with nurses and other health professionals caring for the patient. However, other parties may also claim a legitimate role, such as the patient's family, hospital and managed care administrators, public health authorities, federal, state and local governments regulators, third-party payers, pharmaceutical manufacturers, employers, litigants, police, lawyers, and so on. They may seek information, exercise oversight, establish policies that affect care decisions, offer inducements to provide care in certain ways, and even attempt to dictate care. The justification of the legitimacy of these various claims raises ethical issues.

4.2.2 Family and Friends of the Patient

Traditionally, patients' families have an interest in the care of the patient, and physicians have recognized the legitimacy of that interest. It is common in the specialty of family medicine to say, "The family is the patient." This phrase designates an important strategy of care, recognizing that in all illness, causal and curative factors can be found in the personal relationships that surround the patient. The good physician understands and works with those personal relationships as he or she works with the patient. The role of relatives as surrogate decision-makers was discussed in Section 2.4. They have other roles, such as providing emotional support, giving information, serving as interpreter of the patient's values, or paying the bills. At times, family interests may conflict with the patient's interests: financial concerns or interfamilial disputes may spill into clinical care. Family members may demand forms of treatment that physicians believe are not indicated, or insist on stopping care that is indicated. The cooperation of relatives should be sought and encouraged; at those times when families pose problems about the care of the patient, it is necessary to seek and understand the reasons for their behavior and to attempt conciliation, if possible.

EXAMPLE. An 80-year-old man has severe osteoarthitis and congestive heart failure. He requires constant care and assistance with ambulation. His primary caregiver is his 82-year-old wife, who is in reasonable health, but is troubled with moderately severe asthma. She finds herself unable to provide her husband with the care he requires and encourages him to consider an assisted living facility. He refuses.

COMMENT. Any decision about this gentleman's care is clearly related to his wife's ability and willingness to provide the care he requires. It is clear that interests and medical needs among family members are in conflict. Physicians responsible for the husband's health must be aware that medical decisions are being taken within the context of this conflict. Social work must be engaged to conciliate this conflict and devise mutually suitable arrangements for care.

Different cultures define the role of the family in very different ways. In many cultures, families play a large role in decisions about the patient. This may cause conflicts about appropriate care.

CASE. A Japanese American family brings their maternal grandmother to their primary care physician. Grandmother is 72 years old, came to the United States 10 years ago, and speaks no English. She complains of weakness, weight loss, nausea, and fever of several months' duration. Her grandson, a computer engineer, tells the doctor, "In case you find cancer, we prefer that she not be told. That is the way with our older people. But we do want her to have full treatment." Studies reveal acute lymphocytic leukemia with renal failure, a condition that has a 5% chance for clinical response to aggressive and prolonged chemotherapy.

RECOMMENDATION. In Japanese, and many other cultures, great authority is given to family and especially to senior members, to make decisions about family members. In Topic Two, we stated the major significance of patient's preferences and, at the same time, the importance of respecting cultural values. In this case, we recommend that the patient be informed, through a reliable translator, that she is very sick, that decisions must be made about her care, and then asked whether she wishes to make these decisions for herself or prefers to have them made by another. An authorized delegation of decisional authority instead of simple acceptance of the culture's purported customs is an appropriate compromise.

Singer PA, Viens AM. Religious and cultural perspectives in bioethics [Section IX]. In: Singer PA, Viens AM, eds. *The Cambridge Textbook of Bioethics*. Cambridge, MA: Cambridge University Press; 2009:379–462.

4.2.3 Family Impact of Genetic Testing and Diagnosis

Recent advances in medical genetics, while unquestionably beneficial, introduce many potential conflicts of interest into the care of patients. The principal goals of medicine concern the detection of disease conditions and their causes, followed by appropriate therapy. Usually, diagnosis begins from observation of signs and symptoms in a patient who comes to the physician for advice. However, the rapid development of molecular medicine has generated many tests for the detection of genetic mutations. Some tests have only recently been incorporated into clinical practice; considerable uncertainty about their reliability remains. Many other tests are in commercial development by companies eager to promote their use. The availability of these tests poses many problems to clinicians. In particular, primary care physicians, lacking the detailed knowledge of the genetics and the nature of the tests, may be asked to order a genetic test by a patient anxious about hereditary disease.

These tests are not only done in symptomatic patients to confirm present disease; they can also be done in asymptomatic patients to detect the possibility of future disease. A positive genetic test does not necessarily predict that the person will develop the disease or, if they do, the tests do not predict the timing or severity of the condition. Many diseases known to have a genetic component are currently not amenable to treatment or to preventive measures. Also, genetic tests not only estimate the probability of future disease in the person tested but also the possibly that the mutation is present in the tested person's relatives who share the same genetic heritage. This explains why this section appears in Topic Four rather than Topic One: genetic testing must always be considered within the family context. When a mutation is detected in one member of the family, the question of testing other members may arise. Conflicts of interest between family members, and between the physician and his or her particular patient may arise in genetic testing.

Chadwick R. Genetic testing and screening. In: Singer PA, Viens AM, eds. *Cambridge Textbook of Bioethics*. Cambridge, MA: Cambridge University Press; 2008:160–166.

Lo B. Testing for genetic conditions. In: Lo B, ed. *Resolving Ethical Dilemmas.*
A Guide to Clinicians. 3rd ed. Philadelphia, PA: Lippincott Williams and
Wilkins; 2005:280–285.

CASE. Mrs. Comfort, who was diagnosed with breast cancer at the age of
45 years, suspects a history of breast cancer in her family. She knows
her aunt and her grandmother died of breast cancer. She asks her primary
care physician whether she should be tested for hereditary breast cancer
(mutations in two genes, *BRCA1* and *BRCA2*). She has two adult sisters,
two daughters, age 23 years and 15 years, and one granddaughter, age
2 years. She wonders whether her sisters, daughters, and grandchild should
also be tested.

COMMENT. Primary care physicians may encounter cases such as this one.
Many tests are available on the market and can be ordered. These tests always contain brochures that advise genetic counseling, for which a primary
care physician may not be adequately trained. To ensure adequate informed
consent, pre- and postcounselling with a qualified health care professional,
such as a genetic counsellor is recommended when predictive genetic testing is considered. In considering whether or not to recommend genetic
testing, the following points should be considered:

1. The nature of the genetic disease associated with the mutation, that is,
   the pattern of inheritance (dominant or recessive), the penetrability, the
   variability, and the epidemiologic and clinical course of the disease.
2. The accuracy of the test: its sensitivity, specificity, and predictive value.
3. Options for treatment or prevention of future disease.
4. Implications for one's genetic kinship.
5. Questions of confidentiality, insurance discrimination, and treatment
   availability and access.
6. The educated and informed preferences of the person requesting the test
   and of other persons affected by the results.

RECOMMENDATION. The test for *BRCA1* and *BRCA2* is indicated when a
family pedigree suggests a hereditary breast and ovarian cancer syndrome,
such as a family with multiple individuals with breast and/or ovarian cancer
in several generations, or early onset breast cancer. Mrs. Comfort's family
history is suggestive but the details are not sufficient to confirm this. A
more detailed pedigree might confirm the possibility of a hereditary cancer syndrome and, if present, genetic testing could be considered. If the
patient does test positive for *BRCA1* or *BRCA2* mutations, testing of other
genetically related women should be considered. In addition, those who

test negative without a known mutation in the family, should be counseled that because this particular mutation is only one of the causes of hereditary breast cancer, hereditary breast cancer has not been excluded.

Even individuals who test negative for a known mutation in the family (true negative) are not free of risk: they remain at risk for sporadic breast cancer, which has an incidence of 1 in 8 women in the general population. Preventive options, such as increased surveillance including breast self-examination, mammography, and/or breast MRI or, most drastically, prophylactic mastectomy, must be clearly explained. The predictive genetic testing of minor children for any adult-onset disease is controversial: it is not currently recommended because of the potential to affect the child's view of themselves, the attitude of their parents, and other psychosocial risks. It is advisable to wait until minors are old enough to make the decision themselves. Finally, it should not be assumed that Mrs. Comfort's siblings and other at-risk family members will be interested in being tested or in learning Mrs. Comfort's test results. This must be determined by appropriate inquiry. As molecular medicine advances, many complex ethical problems about obtaining and using genetic information will develop in daily medical practice.

National Cancer Institute Fact Sheet. BRCA1 and BRCA2 Cancer Risk and Genetic Testing. 5.29.09 http://www.cancer.gov/cancertopics. 1/23/2010.

4.3 CONFIDENTIALITY OF MEDICAL INFORMATION

4.3.1 Question Three—What are the Limits Imposed on Patient Confidentiality by the Legitimate Interests of Third Parties?

Information that a patient discloses to a physician is ethically and legally guarded by confidentiality. However, other parties may claim a legitimate interest in that information. Physicians are obliged to refrain from divulging confidential information obtained from patients and to take reasonable precautions to ensure that such information is not inappropriately divulged to third parties. The duty of medical confidentiality is an ancient one. The Hippocratic Oath states, "What I may see or hear in or outside the course of treatment . . . which on no account must be spread abroad, I will keep to myself, holding such things reprehensible to speak about." Modern medical ethics bases this duty on respect for the autonomy of the patient, on the loyalty owed to the patient by the physician, and on the possibility that disregard of confidentiality would discourage patients from revealing useful, but sensitive or embarrasing, diagnostic information. Disclosure may harm the patient or third parties and may encourage use of medical information to exploit patients. Also Federal and state laws stringently limit disclosure (see Section 4.3.2).

Despite these principles and rules, confidentiality is sometimes treated rather carelessly by providers. They may speak about patients in public places, such as hospital elevators or cafeterias; cell phone conversations can broadcast confidential information. Records are not well secured and are accessible to many persons. Technologic developments in information storage, retrieval, and access poses significant problems of confidentiality. Electronic medical records enhance statistical information and facilitate administrative tasks. However, the availability of medical record information to interested third parties, such as employers, government agencies, payers, family members, and others, threatens patient and physician control over sensitive information. For example, the growing use of screening for genetic diseases produces information that may be of interest, not only to patients and their physicians but to the patient's relatives, employers, and insurers. Lack of consensus about how to regulate access to such information poses a continuing problem for health care institutions and policy makers.

Confidentiality is a strict but not unlimited, ethical obligation. Ethically valid claims can be made to gain access to otherwise confidential information. The ethical issue, then, is determining what principles and circumstances justify exception to the rule. The ethical justifications for protecting confidentiality are based on principles of respect for autonomy and privacy of the patient; however, the principle of avoiding harm may limit confidentiality to assure that others are not endangered because they are ignorant of a threat posed by the patient. In general, two grounds for exception to confidentiality exist: concern for the safety of other specific persons and concern for public health.

Beauchamp TL, Childress JF. Confidentiality. In: Beauchamp TL, Childress JF, eds. *Principles of Biomedical Ethics*. 6th ed. New York, NY: Oxford University Press; 2009:302–310.

Lo B. Confidentiality. In: Lo B, ed. *Resolving Ethical Dilemmas. A Guide for Clinicians*. 3rd ed. Philadelphia, PA: Lippincott Williams and Wilkins; 2005: 36–44.

Slowther A, Kleinman I. Confidentiality. In: Singer PA, Viens AM, eds. *Cambridge Textbook of Bioethics*. Cambridge, MA: Cambridge University Press; 2008:43–50.

4.3.2 Health Insurance Portability and Accountability Act

Confidentiality is not only an ethical obligation; it is also mandated by state and federal law. Federal regulations implementing the Health Insurance Portability and Accountability Act of 1996 (HIPAA) create a comprehensive system defining the value, scope, and limits of confidentiality. These regulations are very complex. Most health care institutions have produced explanations of their applicability. Questions about their interpretation should be addressed to the appropriate institutional departments. According to the HIPAA regulations "covered entities," that is, health plans, hospitals, clinics, and health departments, must make a reasonable effort to limit the use and disclosure of individually identifiable information to the minimum necessary to accomplish the purpose of its use or disclosure. Protected health information includes any information, in verbal, written, or recorded form, about a patient that has been received, created, or stored and which includes information that may be used to identify a patient. In general, individually identifiable information obtained by these covered entities should not be used or disclosed without written authorization by the patient.

There are exceptions: clinicians may use and share information necessary for the treatment of patients; the institution may use information to obtain or provide reimbursement or payment for services; the institution may use or disclose information for a variety of policy and assessment activities, such as quality assurance, outcomes, evaluation, etc. Patients also have the right to access their records and, in some cases, to amend incorrect or incomplete information. Covered entities must provide patients with a statement of its privacy policy. Patients are also entitled to receive a list of the situations in which their health care providers and health plans have disclosed their information. Covered entities may be subject to civil and criminal penalties for violations. State laws also exist to safeguard privacy; these may be more stringent than federal law.

In general, the federal regulations do not require the patient's authorization when clinicians must share information for proper treatment. This includes the coordination of care and consultation between clinicians as well as information necessary for referral of patients between providers. Information may also be disclosed to surrogates and family members but only with the patient's consent. It is also permitted to disclose limited information to other inquiring parties, such as friends, clergy, or press. This limited information may include a description of the patient's condition in general terms that do not communicate specific medical information about the patient. The death of a patient may be disclosed by a statement of the fact without further explanation except to authorized persons. Patients, however, may explicitly refuse the release of any information to inquiring parties or limit release to certain persons.

Department of Health and Human Services. Health Insurance Portability and Accountability Act. Standards for Privacy of Individually Identifiable Health Information: Final Rule. 45 CFR Parts 160 and 164:2002.

4.3.3 Confidentiality and Risk to Other Persons

Confidential information may be divulged to appropriate persons when a physician is aware that some identifiable person is endangered by lack of that information. The ethical problem in such cases concerns the probability, nature and seriousness of the risk of harm.

CASE I. A 61-year-old man is diagnosed with metastatic cancer of the prostate. He refuses hormonal therapy and chemotherapy. He instructs his physician not to inform his wife and says he does not intend to tell her himself. The next day, the wife calls to inquire about her husband's health.

CASE II. A 32-year-old man is diagnosed presymptomatically with Huntington's disease. This is an autosomal dominant genetic disease (50% chance of transmitting the gene and the disease to offspring). He tells his physician that he does not want his wife, whom he has recently married, to know. The physician knows that the wife is eager to have children.

CASE III. A 27-year-old gay man is diagnosed as HIV-positive. He tells his physician that he cannot face the prospect that his partner will learn of the infection.

CASE IV. A woman arrives at the emergency department with serious contusions on the right side of her face and two teeth missing. Her nose appears to be broken. Her husband accompanies her. He explains that she tripped on the carpet and fell down a flight of stairs. She affirms his story. The emergency department resident suspects spousal abuse. He does not know the couple, however, and judges by their attire and manner that they appear to be respectable citizens.

RECOMMENDATION. In Case I, the physician should not divulge the husband's diagnosis. While the wife has a moral right to know of her husband's condition, which will certainly affect her deeply, it is her husband's obligation to inform her. The physician, while feeling distressed about the situation, cannot justify disclosure because his legal obligation and his ethical duty to respect his patient's preferences outweighs possible harm to the wife from not knowing her husband's diagnosis. The physician's ethical concerns for the best interests of his patient (as well as the patient's wife) are also relevant. Many physicians would strongly encourage the husband to reveal his condition but should not divulge the diagnosis to his wife. Under HIPPA regulations, the patient has the right to restrict information to any party, including his spouse.

In Case II, a stronger rationale is present for divulging the diagnosis to the patient's wife, namely, the possibility of harm to future children and serious burdens of caretaking that would fall upon her when her husband becomes symptomatic. Serious efforts should be made to convince the husband to seek genetic counseling and to urge him to discuss the matter with his wife. For example, they should explore the use of preimplantation genetic diagnosis and in vitro fertilization. If the wife is also a patient, the physician may encourage her to talk seriously with her husband about his health and their plans for children. Arguments against disclosure are that, although risk of harm to future children is high (50%), the risk is statistical and might not occur. Disclosure will not protect any specific, existing individual. Finally, under HIPAA regulations, the physician is prohibited from disclosing diagnostic information to others. No exception is made for risks to others. The authors believe, that, given the seriousness of Huntington's Disease and the serious burdens it imposes on all parties, disclosure would be the appropriate ethical choice, once all efforts to resolve the issue by counselling have failed. The fact that HIPPA does not explicitly provide for disclosure of risk does not resolve the ethical conflict for physicians. In such a situation physicians may need to seek a legal and an ethics consultation.

In Case III, the physician has a duty to ensure that the partner is informed of his serious risk, first by urging the patient to do so and, if this fails, by taking the steps prescribed in public health law and practice regarding contact tracing and notification. Provisions of local law should be consulted. HIPAA does permit contact tracing and notification if performed in accordance with state and local law.

In Case IV, the resident must make the required report to authorities. The clinical standard for reporting child, spousal, or elder abuse is reasonable suspicion. State laws usually do not allow physicians the discretion not to report. It is the duty of authorized investigators to determine whether abuse has occurred. An emergency department resident should be familiar with the characteristic physical signs of abuse that can frequently be distinguished from other accidental trauma. The apparent respectability of the parties is irrelevant.

4.3.4 Confidentiality and Public Health and Safety

Information obtained from a patient may suggest that he or she might be a danger to others, without identifying specific endangered persons or occasions. Traditionally, certain communicable diseases have belonged in this category, and laws have been enacted that require physicians to report cases of communicable disease to health authorities. Many jurisdictions require persons and sometimes their physicians to report health defects, such as seizures and cardiac diseases, that might render operators of vehicles dangerous to others. Where reporting laws do not exist, and even where they do, ethical problems may arise.

In a precedent-setting case, *Tarasoff v Regents of the University of California* (Cal 1976), a college student informed his psychotherapist that he intended to kill a woman who had rejected his attentions. This threat was not communicated to the woman, whom the student subsequently murdered. The court ruled that the psychotherapist had a positive duty to take reasonable steps to protect third parties from harm, stating "the protective privilege (of confidentiality) ends where the public peril begins." In the opinion of the court, the serious danger of violence to an identifiable person was a consideration that overrode the obligation to preserve confidential information obtained in the course of therapy. It is unclear how this decision would apply to practitioners other than psychotherapists who obtain similar information in the course of providing general medical care. Further, not all jurisdictions accept the Tarasoff rule. Faced with such a situation, a physician would be wise to seek ethics consultation and legal advice.

CASE I. Mr. Cure, with bacterial meningitis, refuses therapy and insists on returning to his college dormitory room.

CASE II. A 28-year-old man who has been under a physician's care for peptic ulcer impresses his doctor as somewhat bizarre in attitude and behavior. The doctor suspects that his patient suffers from a psychotic disorder and asks him whether he is seeing a psychiatrist. He calmly responds that he was once under treatment for schizophrenia but has been well for years. Then, in the course of an office visit, he casually states that he would like to see all politicians dead and was going to attend a political rally "to see what he could do." Should the physician report the patient to the police?

CASE III. A nephrology fellow working in a dialysis unit learns that he is hepatitis C antigen–positive. He approaches another physician, an infectious disease specialist, for advice. After being advised to tell the relevant parties, including the hospital's infection control team, he states that he does not intend to disclose his diagnosis. He insists on confidentiality. Should the infectious disease specialist take steps to have the nephrology fellow's clinical activities restricted?

CASE IV. A 45-year-old woman with a history of idiopathic seizures is diligent about taking antiseizure medication. Her last major seizure was 16 months ago. To qualify for a driver's license, state law requires a physician's declaration that the patient has been free of seizures for 24 months. She pleads with her doctor for this certification because she needs to drive to continue her job.

COMMENT. Most jurisdictions have statutes requiring physicians to report cases of certain types, such as sexually transmitted diseases, gunshot and knife wounds, and suspected child, partner, and elder abuse. The purpose of these statutes is to protect public health and safety, and their ethical justification arises from obligations of social justice. These statutes should be obeyed when the physician believes the legal criteria for making a report are met.

Many jurisdictions have special legislation about confidentiality of HIV testing. The legislation is intended to protect HIV-positive persons from the prejudice that often is directed at them when their condition is known. Usually, this legislation does not permit the testing of persons without their explicit consent and requires their consent to share the results with any other party. Exceptions usually allow other health professionals caring for the patient access to the results and also permit health officers access to the information for the protection of others. Some states have laws that give physicians the discretion to notify sexual partners of HIV-positive persons. Physicians should be aware of the exact provisions of this legislation in their area.

RECOMMENDATIONS. In Case I, bacterial meningitis is an infectious disease. Because this patient's final diagnosis is not clear and could be meningococcal meningitis, which is contagious, spreads rapidly in closed settings, and is a reportable disease, the physician has the duty to communicate the information to college authorities and recommend that Mr. Cure be isolated in the college infirmary, pending the culture results.

In Case II, the danger to others is less clear. No victim is identified, and the likelihood of violence is uncertain. The threat is vague and, as is often the case, possibly empty. Still, the physician should probe for specific details: does he have a particular rally in mind? A particular politician? This patient is obviously in need of psychiatric treatment and should be persuaded to seek it. The consequences to the patient of a police report might be significant. The consequences of reporting "suspicious persons" on the basis of suspicions aroused in medical care might also be socially undesirable. The index for reportable suspicion, in the absence of evidence, should be high; for example, on probing, the patient does state the name of a particular politician and the specific time and place for the rally.

In Case III, the nephrology fellow may infect others and the possibilities for contact are extensive and difficult to limit. "Do no harm" is the premier ethical obligation of physicians. This physician has a direct obligation to protect his patients from harm. If he refuses to do this by reporting himself and by restricting his activities voluntarily, the physician whom he consulted is exempted from confidentiality. She too has a general professional responsibility for the safety of patients. She has a duty to report the nephrologist to the hospital infection control authorities.

In Case IV, the patient is asking the doctor to lie in order to provide a benefit for the patient which may place others at risk. While some physicians are prepared to "bend the law" in cases like these, the safety of the patient herself, of other innocent parties, the integrity of the medical profession, and the utility of the law oblige the physician to refuse her request.

4.4 ECONOMICS OF CLINICAL CARE

4.4.1 Question Four—Are There Financial Factors That Create Conflicts of Interest in Clinical Decisions?

Costs are incurred whenever medical care is provided. Those costs are paid by patients, by their families, by public or private insurers, or they are subsidized by institutions or individuals. Methods of payment are complex, involve many parties, encounter many controls and regulations, and are, in general, opaque to most patients and to many physicians. This complexity provides many opportunities for conflicts of interest and other unfair manipulations. Health care reform debates are centered on this issue. Our book refrains from participating in this complex and difficult discussion. We limit ourselves to payment matters that might directly affect patient care decisions under the present common systems.

The ethical question for practitioners and institutions is how financial arrangments should influence medical decisions in particular cases. How should the legitimate interests of third parties—health care institutions, insurance companies, labor unions, corporations, and government—be factored into clinical decisions about appropriate care? We have seen one example of financial conflict of interest in the self-referral case in Section 4.1.5. Here we explore other related issues.

Some physicians say that these interests should not be factored in and that their only allegiance is to individual patients; societal or institutional costs are not relevant to clinical decisions. Whatever is required by medical indications and personal preferences should be provided. Noble as it is, this view is highly unrealistic. Physicians must consider not only the benefits and safety of an intervention and the patient's preferences, but also its financial implications. This suggests that physicians should be aware of the costs and comparative effectiveness of the diagnostic and treatment proposals that they make to patients. Patients should be informed of the costs so that they can consider this information when deciding which course is best for them. This approach would include, for example, a discussion of the costs of alternative treatments that could be properly recommended for the same treatment. Regrettably, this sort of discussion does not often occur. Physicians rarely know the costs of what they prescribe and order. Even if they do know and disclose this information, most patients are ill-equipped to evaluate medical efficacy in comparision with costs. In the midst of this confused setting, many conflicts of interest arise.

CASE. Dr. S, a 63-year-old physician, suffers from severe, debilitating hip pain due to chronic osteoarthritis. Total joint replacement surgery is covered by Dr. S's insurance plan. His orthopedist knows of a local surgeon who performs innovative microsurgical hip replacements. This procedure offers several advantages over traditional surgery: a smaller incision, no need for general anesthesia, same-day discharge from the hospital, and a shorter recovery period. However, the procedure is new and there is limited outcome data. It is not covered by insurance. Should the orthopedist tell Dr. S about the alternative procedure, even though it performed by a competitor, is innovative, and not covered by insurance?

COMMENT. If the orthopedist does not inform the patient of this alternative, for fear of losing the patient and the fee, the orthopedist has allowed a financial conflict of interest to undermine his obligation of full disclosure. It is up to the patient to decide to seek treatment outside his insurance plan.

If an alternative procedure offers benefits that cannot be realized in any other way, it should be offered the patient.

4.4.2 Health Care Inequities and Clinical Care

In American health care, access and quality vary greatly according to socioeconomic status. Many persons lack insurance or ability to pay for health care and, therefore, have limited access to care. This inequitable structure is often linked to methods of payment to doctors. For example, individual physicians face an ethical problem when they attempt to decide whether they will accept the limited reimbursement from some insurors or restrict their practices largely to well-insured patients.

While individual clinicians are not personally obligated to provide care to the uninsured and underinsured, the medical profession and health care institutions have a moral obligation to work toward justice and equity in health care. Individual practitioners should participate in the planning of their institutions to provide care for the uninsured. Also, individual physicians may provide some service to the underserved, by donating time to free clinics or participating in medical missions.

CASE I. A large, private urban teaching hospital has a policy against providing nonemergency care for uninsured patients. A 55-year-old artist, who is uninsured, is seen in the emergency room for an elevated blood pressure (175/105 mm Hg) and elevated blood glucose (275 mg%). The medical resident in the emergency room would like to provide follow-up care for the patient.

CASE II. A respected and popular internist sets up a boutique practice, inviting his current patients to continue under his care by paying a substantial annual fee. Some of his patients, even those who are insured, cannot afford the fee. Has this physician acted unethically toward those patients?

COMMENT. In Case I, the ethical tension is between the physician's commitment to providing good care for an uninsured patient and the hospital's policy based on financial screening. This is particularly difficult for resident physicians who are employed by the hospital that prevents them from providing needed care. The resident has a confict of interest between his professional role as a healer and his hospital's policy regarding uninsured patients. One resolution is for this resident to find alternative care for this patient, for example, in a free clinic. In Case II, boutique medicine is a form of private practice in which patients pay an annual fee, ranging between several hundred to thousands of dollars, in exchange for round-the-clock access to their personal physician. Boutique physicians accept a relatively small number of patients, enabling the physician to offer increased personal attention, extended clinic visits, and greater accessibility.

Some critics argue that boutique practice is unethical in a health system that fails to provide care for everyone. Boutique practice may reinforce the inequity of the system and, were it to become common, might distort access in favor of the wealthy. Defenders of boutique practice assert that, while it does represent an economic inequality, such inequities are inevitable in a multipayer system. Also, the principle of autonomy dictates that persons should not be limited in what sort of health care they may purchase with their own money. Similarly, physicians should not be limited in their decisions about how many patients to accept or the legal financial arrangements for their acceptance. We believe that boutique practice is not unethical within the present health care system. However, its growth may exacerbate an already inequitable and unjust health care system. Finally, we suggest that it is commendable for boutique practices to admit a certain number of patients whose financial status does not meet the requirements.

4.4.3 Access to Emergency Care and Critical Care

Persons may require immediate care for a life-threatening condition. Some critically ill persons may be uninsured and unable to pay for the care they need. It is an ancient tenet of medical ethics that physicians should provide services in such situations. The Hippocratic writings state, "If there is an opportunity to serve a stranger in financial straits, give full assistance . . . love of humankind and love of the medical art go together" (*Precepts* VI). Most emergency care takes place in hospitals. These institutions operate under various legal requirements that mandate emergency care in certain situations. For example, a federal law (*The Emergency Treatment and Active Labor Act*, EMTALA) prohibits emergency departments from transferring to another institution any patient who arrives with acute symptoms of such severity that absence of immediate medical attention might lead to serious harm. The emergency department must admit and attempt to stabilize a person with a life-threatening condition. This applies also to women who are in active labor. Transfer to another institution is permitted only after such patients are stable, that is, have received treatment necessary to ensure that no deterioration is likely during transfer or that women in labor have delivered their baby. Despite this legal restriction, hospitals may attempt to reduce the financial burden of uncompensated care. Policies developed for this purpose may affect the decisions of physicians working in the institution.

CASE I. A 28-year-old man was brought to the emergency department of a rural hospital after an automobile accident in which he suffered head trauma. He was unconscious, and his wife, who was not severely injured, informed the admitting nurse that they had no insurance. Evaluation revealed a transtentorial herniation and an acute subdural hematoma. The patient was treated with dexamethasone, mannitol, and phenytoin. Because the rural hospital was not capable of providing neurosurgery, an attempt was made to transfer the patient to University Hospital. When it became clear to University Hospital that the patient lacked medical insurance, the transfer was delayed, and the patient died en route to a more distant tertiary care facility.

CASE II. Metropolitan Hospital is located in an urban area where crime and drug use are rampant. Its neurosurgery service is always busy. A large percentage of its patients are uninsured because, in that state, Medicaid eligibility criteria are high (that is, exclude more persons from benefits). Other sources of funds for indigent patients are stretched thin. Still, Metropolitan defines its primary mission as service to its local population, including those who are medically indigent. Although it accepts emergency patients from outlying areas, it requires proof from distant transfers of ability to pay.

RECOMMENDATION. Transfer policies and decisions made in the emergency room must be based on medical indications rather than on financial implications of service in the particular case. It is legitimate for institutions to establish policies that limit the indigent care they provide, but these policies themselves should be consistent with ethical standards and the law. In Case I, the patient's medical indications, requiring immediate neurosurgical intervention, should have met with a prompt response from University Hospital. The solvency of the institution was not at stake. In Case II, the institution attempted to establish a just policy on the basis of a definition of mission in relationship to its prospects for financial solvency. Physicians who work in institutions that receive emergency patients have a communal ethical obligation to ensure that the traditional medical ethic of service to those in urgent need of care can be fulfilled in their institution. Administrators who are physicians and the medical staff authorities should influence hospital policies to this direction.

Beauchamp TL, Childress JM. Allocating, setting priorities and rationing. In: Beauchamp TL, Childress JF, eds. *Principles of Biomedical Ethics*. 6th ed. New York, NY: Oxford University Press; 2009:267–280.
Martin DK, Gibson JI, Singer PA. Priority setting. In: *Cambridge Textbook of Bioethics*. Cambridge, MA: Cambridge University Press; 2008:251–256.

4.4.4 Considering Costs in Clinical Decisions

In recent years, physicians have been urged to consider costs when ordering drugs or procedures. In doing so, they should adhere to certain ethical standards. In general: (a) a physician's first priority should be to provide care that focuses on medical indications and patient preferences. This affirms the physician's responsibility to place the patient's interest before self-interest. Recommendations to patients should be based on best evidence of clinical effectiveness, not on costs to insurers or the institution. Because patients now bear an increasing portion of costs, they have a right to be informed about the expected costs of medicines, tests, procedures, and hospital admissions. They should also be informed of the costs of alternative options that are acceptable.

Some cost-containment measures directly affect the clinical decisions of physicians. Physicians in certain health plans may be encouraged to make clinical decisions about particular patients that are, on the whole, both cost-effective and medically appropriate. This may take the unobjectionable form of merely advising physicians to be "cost conscious," or take the more problematic form of providing incentives, such as bonuses or increased portions of the savings accrued, for physicians who reduce costs. The latter approach results in conflicts of interest that must be conscientiously acknowledged and responsibly managed. It is clearly unethical for a physician to recommend a lower cost but less effective procedure to gain a financial benefit.

CASE I. Mr. S.T., a 52-year-old man with a 3-year history of diabetes and a strong family history of ischemic heart disease, complains to his primary physician of having 3 weeks of exertional substernal pressure. The resting electrocardiogram is normal and a stress test shows ischemic changes in a two-vessel distribution. The patient is treated with aggressive medical management, including beta-blockers, nitrates, statins, and aspirin. The patient improves temporarily but several months later, again complains of chest pain that is sometimes exertional and sometimes not exertional, with a new onset of shortness of breath. At this point, the patient requests a referral to a cardiologist for an angiogram and possible stenting. The physician denies the request because the system in which he practices monitors both quality of care and the appropriate use of expensive referrals, for example, through interventional cardiology. The physician explains his denial by saying that the results of a recent and dependable clinical trial permits continued medical management rather than intervention.

COMMENT. The patient's physician faces a conflict of interest. Her institutional standing is based on practicing high quality care and her salary is based partly on using clinical services appropriately. On the other hand, her professional responsibility is to provide the patient with the best medical recommendations, even if these involve a costly interventional procedure. If the patient had typical exertional chest pain despite maximal medical therapy, the physician would be acting incompetently if she did not recommend a cardiology referral. By contrast, the patient's atypical chest pain while on medical management raises some uncertainty about whether the optimal care for this patient requires immediate cardiology referral.

Ultimately, many of these dilemmas may be resolved by better outcome data. At present, we recognize that in gray areas, where physician practice varies, physicians whose reputation and salary may be at risk, may opt for the least costly alternative. In this case, we believe the physician's judgment, possibly affected by a conflict of interest, is wrong. One large clinical trial (COURAGE) showed that even if medical management is as good as stenting, in general, patients like this one, who develop new cardiac symptoms such as chest pain and new shortness of breath while on medical treatment, require angiogram and stenting.

4.5 ALLOCATION OF SCARCE HEALTH RESOURCES

4.5.1 Question Five—Are There Problems of Allocation of Scarce Health Resources That Might Affect Clinical Decisions?

Scarce resources are distributed by various social mechanisms. Health care in the United States has long been allocated by market processes. The number of physicians, the location of their practices, the ability of persons to pay, and the different perceptions of medical need—these factors and many others result in medical resources being allocated in certain ways. In market allocation, supply and demand are primary factors in distributing resources; some regulations may modify market demand. In recent years, the question has been raised whether medical resources should be allocated by explicit criteria. For example, the state of Oregon established priorities according to which particular treatments for particular disease conditions would be reimbursed by Medicaid. This question belongs to the ethics of health policy and is not discussed in this book. However, any such policy will have effects at the clinical level. Whether physicians should make allocation decisions by balancing societal efficiency against the interests of individual patients will then become a topic for consideration. This is sometimes called "bedside rationing."

CASE. Mr. D.P., a 75-year-old man with a long history of heart disease and diabetes, is admitted to an ICU with fever, hypotension, and shortness of breath. The chest film is consistent with acute respiratory distress syndrome, and the Po_2 is 50 mm Hg. During morning rounds, the intern asks whether aggressive, costly treatment is appropriate for an elderly man who has underlying heart disease and diabetes and whose chances of recovering unimpaired from this episode may be no greater than 35%. At the noon conference, the attending physician asks the house officers whether they should provide indicated treatment or should they begin rationing health care by making tough choices, starting immediately with this elderly man.

COMMENT. The most obvious form of resource allocation for individual physicians—and the least problematic ethically—involves forgoing medical activities that are useless or unnecessary. Costly, scarce resources should not be expended wastefully on patients who will not benefit. Many medical interventions are of this sort. Of course, determining when a particular form of intervention is likely to be useless, unnecessary, or only marginally beneficial requires acute clinical judgment and is often impossible. The recent trend toward outcome studies and clinical epidemiology can be helpful. As illustrated in the case of Mr. D.P., physicians could not be certain when he was admitted whether they were dealing with someone who was "terminally ill" or with a patient who was critically ill but had prospects of full recovery. He subsequently did recover without any impairment. The question raised by the attending about bedside rationing is challenging and provocative. In our view, bedside rationing is not appropriate or ethical. Clinical decisions should be made on the basis of medical indications, patient preferences, and quality of life rather than on societal use of resources unless clear policy guidelines are present, as they are for transplantation (see Section 4.5.5).

4.5.2 Admission to Services with Limited Resources

The entire health care system strains under ever-increasing needs and demands for service. Certain resources, such as funds for unreimbursed care, physician availability, hospital beds, availability of specialty centers, and the like, are *relatively* scarce; that is, the scarcity depends on social or institutional budgets and policy decisions, and are capable of being changed. Other resources, such as solid organs (livers or hearts) are *absolutely* scarce; that is, even with good social policy about their acquisition and distribution, there will always be fewer than needed. Procurement of organs for transplantation exemplifies absolute scarcity. How should health care resources be allocated? This is a policy question beyond the scope of this book. Still, the allocation of scarce resources often directly affects patient care. All commentators on the ethics of this problem agree that resources should be allocated in a fair manner. What constitutes fairness?

It seems fair to establish certain basic objective criteria such as medical condition, potential for benefit, and age, then to select randomly within a pool of those who meet these criteria. Three examples of this problem are medical triage, competing claims for service, and allocation of solid organs.

4.5.3 Triage

Triage is the practice of classifying the sick, injured, or wounded in order to most efficiently employ medical resources in a crisis. Triage on the battlefield is common and generally accepted as ethical. There are rules of triage to establish priorities among wounded soldiers. Triage rules have been applied to other disasters, such as earthquakes and hurricanes. The rules of triage and its rationale are stated in a classic handbook of military surgery:

> Priority is to be given to (1) the slightly injured who can be quickly returned to service, (2) the more seriously injured who demand immediate resuscitation or surgery, (3) the hopelessly wounded may be assigned lower priority for attention. The military surgeon must expend his energies in the treatment of only those whose survival seems likely, in line with the objective of military medicine, which has been defined as "doing the greatest good for the greatest number in the proper time and place."

Emergency War Surgery, NATO Handbook. Washington, DC: United States Government Printing Office; 1958.

COMMENT. The ethical basis for military triage is to return to service those who are needed to fight. Similarly, disaster triage provides priority to persons such as firefighters, public safety officers, and medical personnel in order for them to be returned to rescue work. Also, in epidemic situations, vaccines should be triaged to the most vulnerable and to the necessary providers of care. Present disaster and serious danger to society justify triage rules. Lacking this element of present disaster and the destruction of the fabric of social order, rules that subordinate the needs of individuals to the needs of society are not justified in ordinary clinical situations.

Kayman H, Radest H, Webb S. Emergency and disaster scenarios. In: Singer PA, Viens AM, eds. *Cambridge Textbook of Bioethics*. Cambridge, MA: Cambridge University Press; 2008:281–288.

4.5.4 Competing Claims to Care

There may be regular clinical situations in which personnel, time, equipment, beds, and other factors may be insufficient to accommodate a certain number of patients. Busy hospital emergency departments have a triage nurse who prioritizes patients in view of seriousness of need. However, despite the use of the term *triage* (which means *selection*), the fundamental ethical justification for warfare and disaster triage, namely, contribution to social good, is not present. Rather this is a competition between rival claimants to medical attention.

CASE I. Mrs. C.Z. is a 71-year-old woman who has a diagnosed lung tumor for which she refused surgery. She developed obstructive pneumonia and was admitted to the ICU of the community hospital in her rural county. She has shown no signs of improvement for 7 days. She is now obtunded. The victim of an automobile accident is brought to the hospital with a crushed chest, apparent pneumothorax, and broken bones in the extremities. This trauma patient requires a respirator immediately. Of the six patients on the six respirators in the ICU, Mrs. C.Z. has the poorest prognosis. She seems unable to be weaned and would probably die if ventilatory support were discontinued. Is it ethically justified to recommend to her surrogate that Mrs. C.Z. be removed from the respirator in favor of the accident victim?

COMMENT. The medical prognosis of Mrs. C.Z. is poor. She has cancer of the lung with bronchial obstruction and pneumonia that has failed to respond to treatment. She is comatose and likely to die within days. She is now incapable of expressing preferences. Nothing is known about her preferences, except her refusal of surgery. Given these considerations, the immediate and serious need of an identifiable other person becomes an important consideration. When that person also is in imminent danger of death, the contextual factor of scarcity of resources becomes significant in the decision regarding Mrs. C.Z. In practice, when the resources are only relatively scarce, these situations usually are managed on the scene, by such practices as calling in additional ICU nurses or by making exceptions to the rule about use of ventilators outside the ICU. Such practical stratagems often resolve ethical problems. Should no such solution be possible, we believe that it is ethically permissible to recommend that Mrs. C.Z.'s respiratory support be discontinued.

CASE II. Mr. R.A., the drug addict described in Section 2.5.3 is in need of a second prosthetic heart valve. Several physicians are strongly opposed to providing a second prosthesis. These physicians offer three reasons: (1) surgery is futile, because the patient will become reinfected; (2) the patient does not care enough about himself to follow a regimen or to abstain from drugs; and (3) it is a poor use of societal resources.

COMMENT. The first consideration, futility and the second, noncompliance, are discussed in Sections 1.2.2 and 2.5.2. The third consideration, use of resources, raises the following new ethical issues:

(a) What are the criteria that distinguish good from poor uses of societal resources? Although such criteria might be formulated at the theoretical or the policy level, it is impossible to do so at the clinical level because clinicians do not have an overall view of social need or an understanding of how any particular clinical decision might contribute to that need. Also, attempts to formulate such criteria risk introducing serious bias and discrimination into clinical decisions. As we mentioned earlier, "bedside rationing" is ethically perilous.

(b) There is no guarantee that whatever is "saved" by refusing this patient will be used in any better manner. The societal resources are, of course, not being "absorbed" only by the patient. Instead, they are flowing to the hospital, to the physicians and surgeons, to nurses, and so on.

RECOMMENDATION. The most acceptable ethical justification for refusing to provide a second prosthesis is the medical indication that the risk of surgery with its attendant mortality rate exceeds the risk of managing the patient with medical therapy. Therefore, if medically indicated, the surgery should be offered. Medical indications should not be manipulated as a subterfuge to deny a medically appropriate procedure. A commitment by the patient to enter drug rehabilitation can be a condition of the surgery. The ethical obligation to provide surgical assistance is, however, diminished to the extent that the rights of other patients are directly compromised, as explained in the comment to Case I (Mrs. C.Z.).

4.5.5 Allocation of Solid Organs for Transplantation

In organ transplantation many patients are candidates for absolutely scarce resources. Organ transplantation is a great achievement of modern medicine. For the first time in history, individuals with failure of vital organs such as heart, kidney, and liver can often be saved from certain death by the timely transplantation of a donated organ. In this situation, the organ itself takes on a moral value: its use for one patient makes it unavailable for another. Its use in a less appropriate recipient, and subsequent loss by rejection or the patient's death, deprive a more appropriate recipient of a chance of survival. This represents an unusual "scarce resource": the valuable organ must be given its highest and best use. How does this feature of organ transplant fit into a fair distribution of resources?

The basic ethical principle of organ transplant requires that the organ be a true "donation," that is, a gift voluntarily given by the donor to the recipient. A living donor may make this gift, as is often done between relatives in kidney transplantation and, increasingly, in liver and lung transplantation, or a person may designate that their organs be used after their death, a practice approved by American law. The Uniform Anatomical Gift Act, adopted by all states, provides a system for identification of donors (usually noted on driver's licenses). Ordinarily, organs cannot be retrieved from the dead without prior authorization of the deceased or, after death, by next of kin. Most transplanted organs are obtained from persons declared dead by brain criteria, but in recent years, because the number of deceased donors has remained relatively constant and inadequate, an increasing number of organs are obtained from related or unrelated living donors or from an expanded deceased donor pool that includes sicker and older donors than those previously accepted, as well as and by donation after cardiac death (DCD), sometimes called "nonheart-beating donors". Many state laws require physicians to report impending deaths to the local organ procurement agency which then sends a trained person to request organ donation from the family.

Despite these efforts to increase organ donation, the demand for solid organs far exceeds supply. In the United States in 2008, 27,962 transplants of all organs were performed. At the end of 2008, over 100,000 persons were on the waiting lists for all organs. Of these, 6,601 people died while on the waiting list. Ethical criteria for obtaining and distributing organs must be understood and a fair and equitable system based on these criteria must be maintained. The key elements of such a system are: (1) it avoids social worth criteria; (2) it recognizes the patient's potential for benefit; (3) it has a place for urgency of need; (4) it avoids discrimination on the basis of sex, race, or social status; and (5) it employs a transparent process perceived by the public as fair.

One important feature of fairness is objectivity, based on clinical indicators. In the early days of liver transplantation, allocation relied heavily on the physician's subjective evaluation (degree of ascites, grade of encephalopathy, and need for ICU admission). This subjective system was more susceptible to being "gamed," thus unfairly advancing certain patients to the top of the waiting list. The allocation system has evolved into one in which disease severity is based on objective laboratory criteria (total bilirubin, serum creatinine, and clotting studies). Under the objective criteria, called the MELD score (Model End-Stage Liver Disease) and blood group, a score ranging from 6–40 is assigned to each adult patient on the basis of their expected survival over a 3-month period without transplant. A special weighting of the score applies to patients with hepatopulmonary syndrome, familial amyloidosis, and hepatocellular cancer. These patients are given additional MELD points due to the rapidly progressive nature of these conditions.

Apart from this sort of clinical objectivity, many other factors are necessary for a fair allocation system. In the United States, a government-supported private organization, the United Network for Organ Sharing (UNOS), manages the national list, and local Organ Procurement Organizations (OPO) supervise the distribution of organs. UNOS policy allocates organs on the basis of medical status, blood type, urgency, time on the waiting list, and geographic distance between donor and recipient. A computerized system manages these data. UNOS policies about organ retrieval and distribution can be obtained online.

Lo B. Ethical Issues in Organ Transplantation. In: Lo B, ed. *Resolving Ethical Dilemmas. A Guide for Clinicians.* 3rd ed. Philadelphia, PA: Lippincott Williams and Wilkins; 2005:264–272.

Munson R. Organ transplantation. In: Steinbock B, ed. *The Oxford Handbook of Bioethics.* New York, NY: Oxford University Press; 2007:211–239.

UNOS. http://www.unos.org. 1/23/2010.

Wright L, Ross K, Daar AS. Organ transplantation. In: Singer PA, Viens AM, eds. *Cambridge Textbook of Bioethics.* Cambridge, MA: Cambridge University Press; 2008:145–153.

CASE I. Mr. J.J. is a 50-year-old man with end-stage liver disease caused by primary biliary cirrhosis. He has experienced several complications in recent years, including portal hypertension, bleeding gastric varices, ascites, and one episode of encephalopathy. He has a MELD score of 26. Because the geographic region in which he lives has a long waiting list and because he has a rare blood type, he is unlikely to receive a liver until his MELD score increases to 35. Consequently, at the suggestion of his physician, Mr. J.J. has listed himself at multiple programs in several regions to improves his chance of getting an organ at an earlier stage of his disease.

COMMENT. Taking advantage of multiple listing is not prohibited. UNOS regulations require that patients be informed of the option to multiple list. The question still remains whether multiple listing is fair. Wealthier, better informed, and more mobile patients have distinct advantages in systems that allow multiple listing. This widely used, tolerated, and even recommended way of "gaming the system" introduces discrimination against many patients on the waiting list into a system meant to overcome discrimination. In our view, multiple listing does not resolve conflicts of interest within the organ allocation system, but rather exacerbates it.

CASE II. After two years, Mr. J.J., the patient in Case I, continues to wait for a liver (despite multiple listing). He visits his surgeon's office with a person whom he introduces as "my best friend" and says he has read about some transplant programs that use living donors for segmental liver transplants. Mr. J.J.'s friend says that he would like to volunteer as a living donor. The surgeon has several concerns: (1) Should a healthy person be subjected to the substantial risks of morbidity and mortality associated with donor transplant surgery? (2) Because the surgeon has not performed a living donor procedure, should Mr. J.J. be referred to one of the US programs that has experience in performing such procedures? (3) Can the surgeon verify that this person is really a "best friend" rather than a hired "volunteer" who has agreed to donate for a fee? (4) Should the surgeon do the detective work to determine the truth of the matter?

COMMENT. Although living persons have been kidney donors since the earliest days of transplantation, questions remain about the ethics of doing surgery on a healthy person to benefit another. This practice has been deemed ethical if the donor is an informed, free, and uncoerced volunteer, aware of the risks involved in this operation. Segmental adult liver transplant involves a much higher donor risk than kidney transplantation. Also, obtaining organs by purchase is illegal in the United States and most other countries. It must be very clear that Mr. J.J.'s friend is an informed, free, and uncoerced donor. The surgeon should converse privately with the volunteer, informing him of the risks of the surgery. Federal law requires transplant programs to have a "donor advocate." These advocates explore more deeply the possibility of coercion and medical suitability of donors. Any suspicion of coercion or of financial incentive disqualifies the volunteer. Also, the surgeon should refer the case to a program with ample experience in living donor operations.

4.5.6 Living Unrelated Donors

Case II raises the question about using living, unrelated donors for transplantation. In that case, the problems of possible coercion and illegal donor payment present the primary ethical issues. However, due to the shortage of donors, some transplant programs now accept donors neither genetically nor emotionally related to the recipient. This is known as living, unrelated donation, nondirected donation, anonymous donation, stranger, Good Samaritan, or altruistic donation. Because the ethical basis of transplanation is altruistic donation, there would seem to be no problem with such donors, given their medical suitability. Some transplant services, however, worry that an altruistic act that carries the significant risks entailed by surgery might be the manifestation of a psychiatric condition, and thus not be truly free and uncoerced. (In one major US transplant service, 31% of potential unrelated donors were rejected due to psychological unsuitability.) Careful psychosocial evaluation is ethically imperative.

Another concern is the danger that eagerness to attract nonrelated donors might lead to paying individuals for donating an organ. Transplant organizations have created safeguards in their procurement protocols to avoid this danger. The possibility of commercializing organ exchange is an important reason that organ transplant protocols should remain open and transparent.

Adams PL, Cohen DJ, Danovitch GM, et al. The nondirected live-kidney donor: ethical considerations and practice guidelines: A National Conference Report. *Transplantation.* 2002;74(4):582–589.

Matas AJ, Garvey CA, Jacobs CL, et al. Nondirected donation of kidneys from living donors. *N Engl J Med.* 2000;343(6):433–436.

4.5.7 Donation After Cardiac Death

The usual procedure for obtaining life-sustaining organs requires that death be declared by brain criteria (Section 1.5) prior to removal of the organs. In recent years, a new procedure, called donation after cardiac death or nonheart-beating donation, has been introduced. Although at first controversial, it is now generally considered ethical.

CASE. A 43-year-old woman is brought to the emergency department, somnambulant and disoriented, jaundiced, with asterixis, bruises, and swollen abdomen. She has had 4 days of nausea and diarrhea. Diagnosis is fulminant liver failure due to ingestion of poisonous mushrooms. In the hospital is a 24-year-old man who has been in a vegetative state for 4 months after vehicular trauma. He is ventilator dependant. He has failed three attempts to wean him from the ventilator; he shows no spontaneous respiratory effort. His parents have informed the ICU attending that they are ready to have respiratory support withdrawn. They also have expressed a desire that his organs be donated after death. A physician from the Liver Transplant Service suggests that the patient be taken to surgery where ventilatory support will be terminated and his liver removed for transplant. The ICU attending asks whether this is compatible with the usual rule that organs be removed only after declaration of death by brain criteria.

COMMENT. The practice of nonheart-beating donation does expand the dead donor rule. The patient is taken to surgery, life-support is removed, pain medication is administered, and when the heart stops, death is declared and organ retrieval surgery begins. Ethical criteria for this practice require that the patient be beyond hope of recovery, that permission from designated surrogates be obtained, and that no medications that hasten death be administered. Institutions that utilize this form of organ retrieval should have clear policy, assuring that the practice does not compromise the appropriate care of the donor, that appropriate permissions are obtained, and that all is done in a transparent manner.

Daar AS. Non-heart beating donation: ten evidence-based ethical reommendations. *Transplant Proc.* 2004;36(7):1885–1887.

Institute of Medicine Committee on Non-beating-heart Transplantation. *Non-heart beating organ transplantation: practice and protocols.* Washington, DC: National Academy Press; 2000.

4.5.8 Transplant Tourism

There is brisk international commerce in organs. Available organs and rapid transplantation, often with such amenities as recovery in vacation settings, are advertised on Web sites and through other networks of communication. Clandestine brokers buy organs cheap in poor nations and sell at exorbitant prices to patients in developed countries. The practice of traveling overseas for the express purpose of obtaining an organ transplant is commonly known as transplant tourism. While many overseas transplant centers have technical competence and operate within commonly accepted guidelines for organ procurement, many others are suspect. It is widely known that some organs transplanted at overseas hospitals originate from people who were not able to give informed consent to donation. Some examples are forced donation from prisoners (China), coerced living donation from spouses (India), living donation from those who are uneducated and unable to understand the risks and consequences (India, Pakistan, Philippines), and living donation from the poor who see such as a way of generating income to meet their daily needs (India).

In the United States, all transplant centers have a donor advocate or donor advocate team to ensure safety, welfare, and informed consent of donors. It is not clear that countries outside of the United States have such safeguards for their live donors. In India, for example, many donors suffer significant medical complications and often regret having participated as a donor. Further, the income they have generated by selling their organ in no way removes them from their state of poverty.

Also overseas transplant programs may have looser criteria for accepting patients onto their transplant waiting lists. In the United States, a patient is declined for placement on the organ waiting list when it has been determined that the patient will not benefit from transplant. Patients looking overseas for transplant opportunities should be very cautious about centers promising good outcomes for patients who, actually, may not have good prospects of benefiting from transplant. These unrealistic expectations can also be financially costly to patients and their families.

US transplant teams sometimes encounter patients who have participated in organ tourism, then seek posttransplant care in the United States. This can cause great ethical discomfort for the doctors and nurses.

Sometimes these patients return to the United States with inappropriate immunosuppressant drugs from the foreign hospital. Sometimes they return with complications, such as serious infections (including HIV and hepatitis) and they lack copies of their medical records (or they are written in a foreign language). Documentation of the source of organs is absent.

In the United States, all major transplantation organizations and transplant centers discourage transplant tourism. Often, however, patients desperate for organs will travel for transplant and return home in need of continued or acute care. This poses an ethical problem for domestic transplant centers. They may become complicit in illicit trade, and, most seriously, a patient who needs a retransplant after a failed foreign transplant may use an organ that might otherwise have gone to a patient on the waiting list.

CASE. After 7 years on dialysis, Mr C. notes a Web site that provides access to kidney transplants in Pakistan. The fee required is within Mr. C.'s means. He travels to Pakistan, is lodged in a pleasant hotel, is transplanted with a kidney from a donor unknown to him, and returns home after three weeks. He is now experiencing painful urination and lower back pain. He phones Dr. M., his nephrologist, to schedule a clinic visit. The nephrologist was surprised to learn that Mr. C. had received a kidney transplant overseas and distressed to learn the patient had purchased the organ. The nephrologist's transplant center strongly discourages transplant tourism. Should he accept this patient?

COMMENT. Most advisory policies from transplant organizations discourage accepting such patients, except in emergency situations. However, it seems unfair to reject them if they have previously been a patient. It is advisable to warn current patients against going abroad and inform them that they will not be accepted back if they return with medical problems. It is also advisable to have a list of countries whose laws and regulations about transplant are weak and do not protect their own people against exploitation. Finally, US transplant programs may choose to develop referral relationships with foreign programs where medical competence is high and in countries with organ retrieval policies similar to, if not identical with, American law.

RECOMMENDATION. In the absence of an informed warning about local policy, Dr. M., should accept this patient. He should, however, insist that the local transplant center with which he works develop a policy with the characteristics mentioned in the Comment above for future cases.

4.6 INFLUENCE OF RELIGION ON CLINICAL DECISIONS

4.6.1 Question Six—Are There Religious Issues That Might Influence Clinical Decisions?

Religious belief and the teachings of various faith communities are relevant to medical care. Religion offers powerful perspectives on suffering, loss, and death. The majority of Americans profess some form of religious belief. Also, many persons from other cultures are deeply committed to their religious traditions. Experience reveals the value of religious belief in times of sickness and death. Religious counselors and chaplains have an important role to play in health care. However, Western medicine has long maintained a distance from religion because of scientific skepticism about faith and the professional duty to avoid favoritism toward any religious position. Nevertheless, many physicians respect the tenets of their own religion and allow them to influence their practice of medicine. Catholicism and Judaism both have extensive teachings about health and medical care that may dictate or prohibit certain interventions. However, today persons holding many forms of religious and spiritual beliefs, often unfamiliar to providers, appear in American health care settings. The place of religion in clinical ethics is complex. We have already noted the problems raised for clinical ethics when patients adhere to beliefs that repudiate medical treatment. Here we note some other aspects of religion in clinical care.

Guinn D, ed. *Handbook of Bioethics and Religion*. New York, NY: Oxford University Press; 2006.

Mackler AL. *Introduction to Jewish and Catholic Bioethics. A Comparative Analysis*. Washington, DC: Georgetown University Press; 2003.

Singer PA, Viens AM. Religious and cultural perspectives in bioethics [Section IX]. *Cambridge Textbook of Bioethics*. Cambridge, MA: Cambridge University Press; 2008:379–444.

CASE I. Mr. M.R., a 66-year-old man, has just had a Whipple procedure for pancreatic cancer. His recovery from the surgery has been difficult, and 2 weeks after surgery, he remains in the hospital. His family, Mrs. M.R. and five adult children, are faithfully present in his hospital room. They are all devout Christians. Dr. K., the surgeon, makes rounds twice daily. Each time he comes into the room, the family asks him to pray with them for Mr. M.R's recovery. Dr. K. has no religious affiliation. On one visit, one of Mr. M.R's sons shows Dr. K. an article he has found in the medical literature, claiming that research has shown that patients for whom regular prayer is offered recover more quickly. He reiterates the family's invitation to common prayer.

CASE II. Dr. N.A. is a family practitioner, who also is board certified in obstetrics and gynecology. She is on the staff of a clinic in a neighborhood that has a large population of Ethiopian and Somalian immigrants. Dr. N.A. has earned the trust of women in that community because of her sympathetic understanding of their way of life. She was brought up as an adherent of The Nation of Islam and has studied the Koran and classical Islamic tradition. A delegation of Somalian women visit her and ask whether she will regularly perform ritual genital surgery on the young women of the community. That surgery, technically called clitoridectomy, and referred to by its opponents as genital mutilation, is now done by medically untrained women. Her visitors suppose that she understands that this ritual is required for any devout Muslim woman. Dr. N.A. has seen the medical problems brought on by this procedure. She is repelled by it and knows from her own study of Islamic law that it is not required by the Koran or by the traditions of the prophet.

CASE III. A hospital serves a large population of Hmong immigrants from Laos. Many Hmong people distrust Western medicine and consider surgery, anesthesia, and blood transfusions as dangerous. They have deep trust, however, in the healing rituals of their shamans. The hospital initiated a program to familiarize shamans with medicine and to allow them to perform appropriate rituals for patients.

COMMENT. Although physicians are unlikely to be experts in religious doctrine, they may encounter situations which require them to discuss religious concerns with their patients. Sometimes a physician may choose to refer the family to a more sympathetic colleague or a chaplain. Sometimes, a physician may wish to engage patients and family in a dialogue to learn about their beliefs and to discuss whether those beliefs might affect their care. Such a dialogue should be marked by wisdom, candor, respect, and correct information. Information can be sought from clergy or from other sources The Web site "bioethics for clinicians" of the Canadian Medical Association has a page devoted to this topic (www.cmaj.ca).

RECOMMENDATION. Case I reveals the tension that sometimes arises between accommodating requests from patients and families, and maintaining one's own integrity. If a physician is comfortable joining the family in prayer, it is permissible to do so. It is also permissible respectfully to decline. In this case, the surgeon might tell the family that he will convey their wishes to his colleague physicians and hospital chaplains. He should certainly refrain from any depreciating comments about the scientific quality of studies about the efficacy of prayer in healing.

In Case II, Dr. N.A. is faced with a moral dilemma. She does not wish to lose the confidence of women who badly need a sympathetic physician. Yet, she does not want to see young women mutilated by crudely performed procedures, nor does she wish to be complicit in a ritual that oppresses women. In this case, the weight of the latter concerns should compel her to refuse. She may take this opportunity to begin a respectful dialogue with these women regarding the religious law of their own shared faith and the medical consequences of the practice. Also, it may be asked whether this act constitutes child abuse.

Case III does not represent an ethical problem as such, but a sensitive approach to cultural and religious differences and their impact on health care. The Hmong shamans, Hispanic curanderos, and similar roles in other cultures, are not so much chaplains as practitioners of the healing arts of their culture. As such, they may be excluded from settings where contemporary medicine is practiced. This hospital attempts to incorporate them in a way that is compatible with quality medical care, and complementary to it.

4.7 ROLE OF LAW IN CLINICAL ETHICS

The law has been mentioned many times in this book on ethics. The practice of medicine has long been the subject of legislation, and many judicial cases have involved medical practice, particularly when physicians are accused of negligence. In recent years, the volume of legislation, litigation, and regulation around medicine and health care has increased notably. Although health professionals rarely have detailed knowledge of the law, they should be able to identify potential legal issues and know when to seek legal guidance. For anyone concerned with clincial ethics, certain general knowledge of relevant legal issues is important. For example, topics such as informed consent, confidentiality, advance directives, and many other issues discussed in this book have both ethical and legal aspects.

Bioethics Resources on the Web. Legal Research Resources. http://bioethics.od. nih.gov/legal.html. Accessed November 9, 2009.

Menikoff J. *Law and Bioethics. An Introduction.* Washington, DC: Georgetown University Press; 2001.

4.7.1 Question Seven—What Are the Legal Issues That Might Affect Clinical Decisions?

When ethical conflicts occur in health care, legal rules may sometimes set limits to ethical options or even create ethical conflicts. For instance, a physician may conscientiously believe that she has a moral duty to assist a patient to die by prescribing medications, such as barbiturates, so that the patient may take his own life. The laws in her state, however, prohibit medically assisted dying by making it a crime for physicians to provide the means. Health professionals may sometimes feel conflicted between the ethical duty to protect confidential communication and legal duties to make required reports to protect public health or safety. In general, codes of professional ethics impose upon professionals the duty to obey the law. Physicians may sometimes feel frustrated by laws that seem burdensome, such as reporting requirements or the elaborate restrictions of HIPAA on communication of patient data. Physicians occasionally falsely believe or assert that the law imposes duties that are not required. Also, some physicians have an inordinate and uninformed fear of liability. Studies have shown that physicians may seek legal information from highly unreliable sources, namely, from other physicians.

McCreary SV, Swanson JW, Perkins HS, Winslade WJ. Treatment decisions for terminally ill patients: physicians' legal defensiveness and knowledge of medical law. *Law Med Health Care.* 1992;20(4):364–376.

We have stated summary positions of federal and state laws, as well as judicial decisions at the points where we treat particular ethical issues, such as forgoing life support in Section 3.3.7. When reference to these and other legal standards arise in clinical ethics, it is crucial to distinguish their relevance to the case under discussion. Often, circumstances of the legal case differ importantly from the case at hand. Laws of one state do not apply in others; judicial decisions of one jurisdiction may or may not be relevant in another. If a legal question presents itself in a clinical ethics case, it is prudent to seek advice from persons knowledgable about law in bioethics. Possession of a legal degree does not guarantee familiarity with law in bioethics. Hospitals should be sure that its legal counsel has this competency and that its risk management division is similarly competent. Hospital ethics committees should be able to identify, among its own members or elsewhere, suitable advisors about the law.

A common fault is to allow a discussion of the law to preempt an ethical discussion. Although legal issues may be relevant to the case, they rarely settle ethical problems. Ethical problems must be analyzed by ethical concepts and reasoning, as this book illustrates.

4.8 CLINICAL RESEARCH

Clinical research is essential to modern medicine: new therapeutic and diagnostic interventions must be tested and evaluated by applying them to humans, and often those humans must be patients, persons suffering from the disease for which the intervention is designed. In the past, patients were often unwilling and unknowing subjects of clinical research. Today, this is ethically and legally unacceptable, and research is clearly distinguished from treatment. Physicians should know how that distinction is made and be aware of their responsibilities when they undertake clinical research. Until recently, most research was done within academic hospitals by trained investigators; today, pharmaceutical companies invite many practitioners to participate in research protocols by enrolling their patients in a clinical trial. Many of the practitioners may have had little research training and may be unfamiliar with the ethical requirements of research. Clinicians should assure themselves that any protocol that they are invited to join has been properly reviewed in accord with federal regulations. Ethics training for investigators is required by the National Institutes of Health.

Beauchamp TL, Childress JF. The dual roles of physician and investigator. In: Beauchamp TL, Childress JF, eds. *Principles of Biomedical Ethics*. 6th ed. New York, NY: Oxford University Press; 2009:317–324.

IRB: Ethics and Human Research. Garrison, NY: The Hastings Center. http:// thehastingscenter.org/Publications/IRB. Access date 1/23/2010.

Levine RJ. *Ethics and Regulation of Clinical Research*. New Haven, CT: Yale University Press; 1988.

Lo B. Clinical research. In: Lo B, ed. *Resolving Ethical Dilemmas. A Guide for Clinicians*. 3rd ed. Philadelphia, PA: Lippincott Williams and Wilkins; 2005:176–184.

Singer PA, Viens AM. Research ethics [Section V]. *Cambridge Textbook in Bioethics*. Cambridge, MA: Cambridge University Press; 2008:185–240.

4.8.1 Question Eight—Are There Considerations of Clinical Research and Education That Might Affect Clinical Decisions?

It is commonly recognized that research itself involves many conflicts of interest. But the most obvious clinical–ethical issue is that clinical research constitutes an intrinsic conflict of interest when the clinician is also a researcher. A clinician–researcher has an obligation to particular patients and an obligation to perform accurate research according to protocol. These two duties may occasionally conflict. Also, research often includes normal subjects, who are not patients of the physician–researcher. The question is whether that normal subject, once under the observation of the researcher, is constituted a sort of patient, to whom the researcher has responsibilites similar to those toward regular patients?

4.8.2 Definition of Clinical Research

Clinical research is defined as any clinical intervention involving human subjects, patients, or normal volunteers, performed in accordance with a protocol designed to yield generalizable scientific knowledge. The protocol states the research techniques, such as randomization and double blinding, as well as the statistical techniques necessary to establish validity of the data. The benefits of research accrue to persons other than the subject of research, namely, to future patients, to the professional doing the research, and to the society in general. Even when the subject personally benefits—for example, a cancer goes into remission as the possible result of treatment with an experimental drug—future patients benefit from the knowledge produced by the research. The research protocol is usually designed as a clinical trial in which patients are randomized between the investigative intervention and an alternative, such as a placebo or current best treatment. This randomization is ethically justified by "clinical equipoise," that is, the opinion of the relevant community of experts that, on the basis of available evidence, there is no known difference between the trial intervention and alternatives. The purpose of the research is to demonstrate that this assumption is correct or is wrong in favor of one or the other treatment. In addition, patients and usually investigators are not aware of which intervention the research subject is receiving.

London A. Clinical equipoise. In: Steinbock B, ed. *The Oxford Handbook of Bioethics*. New York: Oxford University Press; 2007:571–596.

4.8.3 Regulation of Clinical Research

Clinical research is guided by ethical principles promulgated in several statements, principally the Nuremberg Code, the Helsinki Declaration of the World Medical Association, and the Belmont Report, the prologue to the US Federal Regulations. These federal regulations, promulgated by the US

Department of Health and Human Services, state precise rules that govern all research done in institutions that receive federal funds and also any research done in private industry that will be submitted for FDA approval. The following actions are required by these regulations:

(a) Review of proposed research by an Institutional Review Board (IRB). These boards are usually situated in universities and research institutions, although today there are commercial IRBs, authorized by the government to review research from private investigators. The IRB consists of persons competent to understand the science of the protocol and other informed persons, some of whom should be independent of the institution. This IRB reviews the protocol and recommends approval or disapproval to the funding agency. The ethical issues regarding research must be resolved in the course of the review, for example, an appropriate risk–benefit ratio, the details of informed consent, and the suitability of compensation to subjects.

(b) The IRB must ascertain that recruits are provided accurate information about the research purposes, procedures, and risks. This information must stress the voluntary nature of participation in research and indicate that the patient's refusal to participate will not compromise the care and attention due to all patients. It is important to avoid "therapeutic misconception," that is, implying that the research is some form of treatment beneficial to the patient, and that "new" means "better." Coercion, due to excessive compensation or to the professional authority of the researcher, must be avoided. Investigators should document their efforts to assure that research subjects understand and consent to the conditions of the protocol.

(c) IRBs must assure the fair selection of subjects. Attention must be paid to the selection of appropriate populations as research subjects; that is, researchers must avoid taking advantage of vulnerable populations. Vulnerable populations, such as children, mentally incapacitated persons, and prison inmates, are identified in the federal regulation. Special regulations apply to their participation; they are sometimes excluded as research subjects. Investigators must seek to achieve racial and gender balance, to the extent compatible with the objectives of the protocol.

45 Code of Federal Regulations 46:1981; 48:1983.
Sugarman J, Mastroianni AC, Kahn JP, eds. *Ethics of Research with Human Subjects. Selected Policies and Resources.* Frederick, MD: University Publishing Co; 1998.

4.8.4 Innovative Treatment

While new drugs and devices must undergo testing before being marketed, medicine involves much more than drugs and devices. New approaches to diagnosis and treatment are constantly evolving. Some of these may be tested in formal reasearch but many will be tried by individual physicians before any formal determination of this utility. Physicians may use FDA-approved drugs "off-label" to treat conditions beyond those for which the drug was approved. Surgeons, in particular, may modify or create entirely new surgical maneuvers.

COMMENT. This is called *innovative treatment*. Clinicians may use such methods in the care of a particular patient. They should do so prudently, with solid conviction that the new use or procedure is likely to be safe and effective. Innovative treatment is not, as such, governed by the codes and regulations that govern research. However, it should be governed by the same spirit. The advice of knowledgeable colleagues should be sought; a risk–benefit ratio as accurate as possible should be worked out; and the consent of the patient to be the recipient of yet untried treatment should be obtained. If a clinician believes that innovative treatment might be generalized into standard practice, it is advisable to formulate a properly designed research project. In doubtful cases, clinicians should seek the advice of the IRB about the advisability of innovative treatment and about whether such treatment should be provided only in a properly designed and reviewed protocol. Misjudgment in using innovative treatment can lead to malpractice charges.

Investigational treatment describes forms of diagnosis and therapy that are under development and have not reached the stage where a formally designed clinical trial has demonstrated efficacy. Existing data suggest that the treatment is "promising." Patients suffering from a condition for which no effective therapy exists may seek such treatment, and their physicians, even if skeptical about its efficacy, may be eager to offer hope. Third-party payers usually explicitly exclude investigational (sometimes called "experimental") treatment from coverage and managed care organizations typically discourage its use. However, some insurers and health care organizations are willing to consider payment for investigational treatments that are promising, on a showing of clinical appropriateness.

EXAMPLE. Hematopoietic stem cell transplantation is rapidly developing as a standard therapy for many hematologic malignancies. Allogeneic stem cell transplantation from HLA-matched donors has curative potential for relapsed Hodgkin's and non-Hodgkin's lymphoma, relapsed and high-risk initial acute myelogenous and lymphocytic leukemia, and multiple myeloma. Remission has been effected in other conditions, such as chronic myelogenous leukemia and aplastic anemia. However, it is still considered experimental for many other conditions, such as primary amyloidosis, myelodysplastic syndromes, and some solid tumors, such as kidney cancer. Bone marrow transplant is often viewed as a last hope in refractory disease. When patients face an almost certain death from their disease, they may be willing to accept the high risk of death associated with experimental bone marrow transplantation.

COMMENT. Investigational treatments should be recommended with great caution. Their promise is often unfulfilled, and their negative effects are often underestimated. At the same time, patients may have no other recourse and medicine advances by these tentative steps. Physicians should make every effort to ensure that their patients see both the risks and benefits in a realistic light. Administrators of health plans should formulate clear policies on provision and reimbursement for investigative procedures and establish means of assessing such treatment. In the 1990s, reports of favorable results from high-dose chemotherapy followed by stem cell transplant for advanced breast cancer prompted many women and their doctors to seek this highly investigative and highly risky procedure. Pressure from patients and from judicial decisions forced insurers to cover the procedure. When investigative studies were completed, it became clear that the procedure offered no advantage over standard treatment and had much higher adverse effects. Thus, the hope of many patients for cure or remission ended in disappointment. Some deaths may have been hastened by the procedure.

4.8.5 Compassionate Use of Investigational Drugs

While a drug is being studied in an approved research protocol, a physician may determine that, even though data do not yet confirm its efficacy and safety, it may be the only available treatment for the patient with an immediately life-threatening disease. The FDA has a provision to allow the physician and the sponsor of the new drug to petition for its use in treatment. This is commonly called "compassionate use" (although the FDA does not use this term). The physician must demonstrate a reasonable basis for believing that the drug may be effective, that its use would not expose the patient to significant additional risks, and that there is no satisfactory alternative drug. The sponsoring company must affirm that it is actively pursuing marketing approval of the drug.

4.8.6 Ethical Problems in Clinical Research

All clinician–researchers should honor the ethics of clinical research by adhering to the requirements of informed consent of subjects and review of protocols by competent bodies, such as IRBs. Above all, they must be aware of the intrinsic conflict of interest between their duties to their patients and responsibility to the research protocol. It might be asked whether a particular patient, who is in general an appropriate candidate for an approved protocol, should be approached because the risk–benefit ratio is questionable in this patient's case. This problem might arise in situations in which a new drug, believed to be of potential benefit from preliminary animal and human investigations, is compared in a formal clinical trial with a placebo. In double-blind trials, neither the doctor nor the patient knows whether the patient is receiving a drug or placebo. Some physicians find this situation clinically and ethically unacceptable. Some physicians are concerned that their patients may be randomized to an inferior therapy. It can be asked whether patients should be continued on protocol, or new patients entered, when a clinician–researcher believes the majority of patients whom he has treated seem to benefit from one experimental drug rather than the standard treatment.

EXAMPLE I. A clinician is entering patients in a randomized double-blind trial of a drug to prevent angina. He suspects from the side effects which is the standard drug and which is the experimental one. He also has the impression that patients are doing much better on the suspected research drug than on the standard one.

COMMENT. The investigator seems caught between two obligations: the duty to benefit his patient and the contractual duty to carry out the trial. In principle, the duty to benefit the patient supersedes all other duties. Only if the investigator is convinced that the use or nonuse of a test drug may cause harm does it become unethical to proceed. However, in this situation, suspicion and clinical impression should not override scientifically founded uncertainty until properly collected data are analyzed. Soundly designed clinical trials should have oversight mechanisms (such as planned interim analysis and data safety monitoring boards) to monitor trends, to deal with occasional clinical impressions, and to terminate the trial, should the evidence of distinct benefit or harm become persuasive.

EXAMPLE II. A new drug is being tested to determine its efficacy in treatment of cytomegalovirus (CMV) retinitis, a frequent infection of persons with AIDS and one that can result in blindness. A strictly controlled trial has been designed to gather the most valid data possible, because the known adverse effects of the drug must be balanced by demonstrated benefits. One aspect of the controlled trial is a random allocation of patients into two groups, one of which will receive the new drug and the other a combination of the two best currently used drugs. A physician involved in the trial finds that certain of her patients specifically request the new drug on the grounds that an AIDS advocacy Web site declares that it is more effective in preventing blindness. She wonders whether she should provide the drug outside of the controlled trial.

RECOMMENDATION. This is not an instance of compassionate use because other treatments are available (see Section 4.8.5) The investigator should not provide the drug outside the trial. The trial is based on the hypothesis that the new drug and the old drugs are equivalent; the outcome of the trial will demonstrate the superiority of one over the other, on the basis of clinical efficacy and drug toxicity. In the absence of final or convincing data, the investigator should disabuse those who seek the experimental drug of the idea that it will give them a better chance. Use of the drug outside the trial will confound the evidence necessary to demonstrate the effectiveness of the new drug. Also, as in the treatment of advanced breast cancer mentioned earlier, its use may cause direct harm to patients.

CASE III. The investigator of the cytomegalovirus drug trial is a paid consultant of the sponsoring pharmaceutical company and holds several hundred shares of the stock.

CASE IV. In 1999, Jesse Gelsinger, an 18 year old with ornithine transcarbamylase deficiency, died while participating in a gene therapy trial. His disease had been well controlled by diet and medication. His motivation for volunteering was to advance science and help patients suffering from the same disease. After his death, it was revealed that the principal investigator was an investor in the company that sponsored the trial. Gelsinger had not been informed, when he volunteered, about certain serious adverse effects that had already occurred in the trial; similar effects were the cause of his own death.

COMMENT. Conflict of interest occurs when an investigator may benefit financially from the outcome of a trial. This incentive may influence choice of research subjects, adequacy of consent (as in Gelsinger's case), or analysis of data. A researcher with financial interests at stake has an incentive to modify the results of the trial, either by falsifying data or by interpreting ambiguous data to favor the trial drug. Although conflicts have always existed in scientific investigation—a Nobel prize, a promotion, a publication—in recent years financial interests have loomed large. Investigators may become founders of research companies, have significant holdings, are compensated for their scientific advice or their lecturing on behalf of products. Policy statements from government and professional organizations now recommend that any such conflict of interest should be disclosed to research subjects (Gelsinger was not informed).

RECOMMENDATION. Policies, regulations, and the requirements of most research institutions insist that investigators take the following actions: (1) disclose their financial interests to the institution and even to the research subject; (2) identify their financial affiliations in any published papers; (3) divest themselves of substantial interests; (4) participate in mechanisms to ensure the validity of data, such as outside peer review. Even when such rules do not exist, these actions have moral cogency. Physicians who have involvement with drug sponsors should recuse themselves as investigators for the products of those companies.

This case also raises the question mentioned earlier: to what extent does a research subject become a patient of the investigator? Jesse Gelsinger was not under the care of the investigator when he volunteered for the trial. We strongly advise that the role of researcher and the role of clinician should be carefully distinguished. However, all research subjects are under supervision and observation by clinician–researchers. Major codes of research ethics state the priority clearly: "the health of my patient will be my first consideration" (*Declaration of Geneva*, WMA) and "Concern for the interest of the subject must always prevail over the interests of science and society" (*Physician's Oath*, WMA). It seems clear that if an investigator perceives that the research procedure may have serious adverse effect, he or she assumes a physician role toward that research subject. That role begins with a recognition of the subject's condition, taking immediate steps in an emergency situation. At that point, the considerations mentioned about withdrawal of subjects from a study (see Section 4.8.6) become pertinent. An outside physician should take over any necessary continuing care.

Association of American Medical Colleges. Protecting Subjects, Preserving Trust, Promoting Progress. Policy and Guidelines for the Oversight of Individual Financial Interests in Human Subjects Research. October 2002.

Department of Health and Human Services. Financial Relationships and Interests in Research Involving Human Subjects. March 2003.

4.9 CLINICAL TEACHING

Many patients receive care in institutions where clinical teaching is done. Their disease and its diagnosis and treatment provide an opportunity for students in the health sciences to learn the skills of practice. Often, treatment will be provided by a student. Naturally, proper oversight is ethically imperative. However, it is possible that some clinical decisions are made with a view to teaching and that such decisions may conflict with the patient's interests and/or wishes.

Lo B. Ethical dilemmas students and house staff face. In: Lo B, ed. *Resolving Ethical Dilemmas. A Guide for Clinicians*. Philadelphia, PA: Lippincott Williams and Wilkins; 2005:226–234.

4.9.1 Consent to be a Teaching Subject

Upon entering a teaching hospital, patients usually sign a general consent to participate in the teaching enterprise. Many patients, particularly those who are seriously ill at the time of admission, or who, for other reasons, cannot comprehend the meaning of the teaching hospital consent form, have probably not given adequate informed consent to be used as teaching subjects. Most persons who are admitted to a teaching hospital have little or no understanding of what it means to be cared for in such an institution. They do not know the different levels of their providers' education and training. They are unaware of the possible tensions between training new clinicians and providing quality care.

Patients should be asked specifically about each episode of teaching and invited to participate. Consent should be tailored to the diverse levels of risk entailed when procedures are done by a student and by an experienced clinician. The fact that a particular procedure will be done by a student, and that it is for teaching rather than for their care or in addition to their care, should be made clear. Students should identify themselves as students and politely request the patient's permission to do a procedure. Refusal should be accepted graciously.

For purposes of the medical school course on history taking and physical diagnosis, many patients provide their histories to five or more students and allow their bodies to be probed without complaint. It is particularly important that, when the occasional patient refuses to participate in one or another teaching exercise, the student and the faculty respect the patient's wishes absolutely and not threaten or intimidate the patient in any way. Medical students and physicians must remember that individual patients are not obligated to participate in the training of society's future physicians. Yet, they almost invariably are eager to do so. Clinical teachers and students should be grateful for patients' generosity.

In teaching hospitals, relatively inexperienced students perform many procedures, including blood drawing, intravenous insertions, lumbar punctures, paracenteses, thoracenteses, and occasional endotracheal intubations. Students must be supervised by attendings, residents, or senior nurses as they learn these procedures. Students often remark (in private) about their feelings concerning these procedures. They are eager to learn these skills and believe they must master these techniques to function effectively as physicians. Still, they are not sure how to approach the patient and how much disclosure is appropriate for the patient's informed consent, particularly for relatively innocuous, albeit discomforting, procedures, such as venipuncture.

CASE I. A 52-year-old obese woman required a lumbar puncture. She had signed a consent form for teaching procedures. A second-year resident entered her room with two medical students. He told the patient that she needed a procedure, positioned her and, when she was turned toward the wall, handed the syringe to the medical student, indicating that she was to draw spinal fluid. The student had seen the resident perform the procedure on the previous day. The resident then left the room. After several unsuccessful attempts, one medical student sought the resident who, on returning, said, "You've got to learn!"

COMMENT. This case is not an ethical problem; it is an ethical outrage. No consideration was shown to the patient's feelings, appropriate informed consent was not obtained, supervision was inadequate, and easily arranged accommodations were not made. Students are often offended by being placed in such situations. As low persons in the medical school hierarchy, students may feel an ethical conflict and not know how, and to whom, to express their feelings (see moral distress discussed in Section 4.1.4.)

Any senior person who orders a student to perform a clinical procedure assumes responsibility for the safe execution of the procedure and for its consequences. They should remain present when inexperienced students make their early attempts. Senior persons should invite students to express their discomfort or doubts about what they are asked to do. We must note that the case above appeared in the first edition of this book in 1982. We have subsequently inquired of medical educators whether it is still pertinent. The answer is inevitably "yes."

CASE II. A 74-year-old man with diabetic ketoacidosis is admitted in coma and profoundly dehydrated. The patient requires large amounts of fluid and doses of insulin. A peripheral IV line is placed. The chief resident suggests a central venous catheter be inserted. One of her reasons for this decision is to allow an inexperienced intern to practice this technical procedure.

COMMENT. Procedures involving any risk should be performed only for diagnostic or therapeutic purposes. Risky procedures should never be done exclusively or even partially for their teaching value. In Case II, the intern's need for additional practice should not affect the chief resident's clinical judgment. If the procedure is harmless, such as palpation or auscultation, or involves only minor inconvenience, such as asking a patient with ataxic gait to get up from a chair and walk across the room, or minor discomfort, such as extension and flexion of an arthritic limb, patients may be requested to allow the procedure. Noninvasive procedures, involving neither risk nor discomfort, such as auscultation or examination of pupils or skin, are permitted even on patients who lack decisional capacity.

CASE III. A second-year medical student is being mentored by a surgeon in private practice. A 22-year-old woman has been prepared for an appendectomy and is now under anesthesia. The surgeon suggests that the student might do his first pelvic examination on the unconscious patient.

COMMENT. This is ethically unacceptable. The patient has not consented to this particularly intimate procedure and, even though unconscious, suffers an offense to her dignity and a violation of the patient–physician contract. The student is embarrassed, both at doing the examination and at expressing his discomfort to his mentor. Medical schools should have careful guidelines on this subject and, if possible, arrange teaching experiences that are acceptable to students and to patients.

Christakis DA, Feudtner C. Ethics in a short white coat: The ethical dilemmas that medical students confront. *Acad Med.* 1993;68(4):249–254.

4.9.2 Teaching Procedures on the Newly Dead

Many teaching programs use the cadavers of newly dead patients to teach various nonmutilating procedures, including tracheal intubation, placement of central venous catheters, and pericardiocentesis. In one study, only 10% of the programs that used newly dead patients for teaching obtained either verbal or written consent from the patient's survivors. Proponents of training on the newly dead argue that it is beneficial to society, does not mutilate the cadaver, and that no good alternatives are available. They further argue that consent need not be sought because consent can be presumed for harmless procedures and because the grieving survivors should not be further troubled about something that is not harmful or mutilating to their deceased relative. It is our opinion that, although the newly dead may be used to teach some procedures, it is ethically obligatory to seek consent from next of kin. This acknowledges that we recognize and respect the special status of the newly dead person; omitting consent is a violation of trust. Many families have religious or cultural beliefs that should be respected. Also, secretive activities are offensive to many health professionals, including medical students and nurses. Finally, a number of studies have shown that consent for procedures, such as endotracheal intubation, can readily be obtained from family when they are approached in a sensitive and respectful manner.

4.9.3 Autopsy

Autopsy is performed on cadavers of the newly dead, often for teaching purposes. Once routine, it is now performed only in certain situations. Coroner's rules require autopsy when the cause of death is uncertain. Otherwise, autopsy requires permission of the family of the deceased. It is generally known that Judaic and Islamic traditions prohibit mutilation of the cadaver, but less generally appreciated that these traditions allow certain exceptions, particularly if the information gained from the autopsy contributes to the life and health of others. Consultation with religious authorities about these rules is advisable. Families should be approached with particular sensitivity.

4.10 PUBLIC HEALTH

4.10.1 Question Nine—Are There Issues of Public Health and Safety That Affect Clinical Decisions?

Public health is the science and practice of preventing disease and promoting health in populations. As a science, it depends largely on epidemiology and, as a practice, is usually performed by governmental organizations, such as the Centers for Disease Control and Prevention, the Public Health Service, and local health departments. The traditional objectives were the control of communicable disease, the safety of the water and food supply, and response to natural disasters. More recently, public health has turned to broad educational efforts to enhance the health of the public by warning of health risks, informing about healthy lifestyles, and encouraging preventive care, such as prenatal monitoring. Since September 11, 2001, public health authorities have been called upon to deal with bioterrorism attacks and have been asked to develop plans to deal with biologic, chemical, and nuclear threats. Many of the ethical issues of public health are matters of policy and are beyond the scope of this book. However, public health intersects with clinical care at several points. The protection of the public from communicable diseases, for example, is occasionally in conflict with the medical duty of confidentiality. This is discussed in Section 4.3.3. One aspect of public health, the immunization of children, is a particular issue for pediatric ethics.

Faust HS, Upshur R. Public health ethics. In: Singer PA, Viens AM, eds. *Cambridge Textbook of Bioethics*. Cambridge, MA: Cambridge University Press; 2008:274–281.

Lo B. Ethical issues in public health emergencies. In: Lo B, ed. *Resolving Ethical Dilemmas. A Guide for Physicians*. 3rd ed. Philadelphia, PA: Lippincott Williams and Wilkins; 2005:280–285.

4.10.2 Occupational Medicine

Physicians may practice within institutions whose functions and structures may conflict with the physician's allegiance to patients. For example, military phyicians, prison or police physicians, and physicians working for industry may encounter conflicts of interest. As physicians, they are obliged to serve those who come to them for care; as employees, they also have obligations to the organization. Ethical problems, particularly about confidentiality may arise.

CASE. A worker in an industry using potentially harmful chemicals visits the company physician about a persistent cough. The physician does a cursory physical and prescribes a cough medicine. It is company policy not to investigate symptoms of this sort too aggressively until they become demonstrably more serious. It is also policy not to suggest to worker–patients the potential for lung disease or to make employee health records available to them.

COMMENT. The company policy is manifestly unethical because it causes persons who may be benefited by early diagnosis and treatment to be deprived of it through remediable ignorance. The physician who accepts such a policy clearly acts unethically, because duties to patients are disregarded without the patients being made aware of the physician's dual role. The Code of Ethics of the American Society for Occupational Medicine requires physicians working in such settings to "avoid allowing medical judgment to be influenced by any conflict of interest" and "to accord highest priority to the health and safety of the individual in the work place." This implies that conflicts should be resolved in favor of individual patients, even if this is to the detriment of the company and the physician. Physicians accepting positions with dual responsibilities should be certain that their employers will allow them to abide by the ethical code.

A most serious ethical problem may challenge physicians and other health professionals during wartime. They may be ordered to participate in "enhanced" interrogation techniques, not as agents but to assure that these techniques, which are highly dangerous, do not cause death or serious injury. It is our opinion that such activity is a most serious violation of ethics. Torture, or any procedure that approaches it, aims to destroy the dignity, self-respect, and autonomy of its victim.

Singh A. Physician participation in torture. In: Singer PA, Viens AM, eds. *Cambridge Textbook of Bioethics*. Cambridge, MA: Cambridge University Press; 2008:350–358.

4.10.3 Physicians' Duty During Epidemics

Professional ethics require physicians to place their patients' interest above their own. In times of an epidemic, many of the sick and potentially sick are not "patients" of individual physicians. What are the duties of physicians toward the sick in such situations? This is an ancient question, now revived as new and dangerous communicable diseases appear in epidemic form. During the historical debates over the physicians' duty, no consistent view emerged: some commentators argued for a stringent duty to care for the sick even at risk to self; others viewed this service not as a duty but as an altruistic action and allowed for many exceptions; still others recommended flight and avoidance.

COMMENT. Physicians have long accepted that infection from their patients and work setting is an occupational risk. They are aware that precautions must be taken. At the same time, the duty to preserve health and protect family, with the corresponding right to do so, is legitimate. The extent of this duty must be evaluated with respect to the nature, probability, and seriousness of the risks, alternative strategies, the infringement on others' rights, and the social consequences of various courses of action.

When HIV/AIDS first appeared in the 1980s, this ancient debate was renewed. Because the physician's duty was widely discussed, we use that debate as an example of the duty to provide care during an epidemic. A similar analysis must be made for each infectious agent (and can often be obtained from CDC Web sites). In summary, the HIV/AIDS debate taught the following lessons.

(a) It is crucial to develop accurate information about the incidence of infection, disease, and mortality. For health professionals in general, the danger of HIV infection by contact with a patient is low, but not negligible. The risks for orthopedic surgeons, given the nature of their work, is probably somewhat greater than for other surgeons and considerably greater than for physicians who do not have regular contact with bodily fluids. Risk of infection is related to the potential for percutaneous exposure to blood. Hollow-bore needle sticks pose the greatest risk to health professionals. Nurses, phlebotomists, house officers, and medical students are the groups at greatest risk. After a hollow-bore needlestick, risk of HIV infection appears to be low—about 0.3% overall. Further, postexposure prophylaxis with azidothymidine effectively reduces the transmission rate, by 79% according to one study.

Centers for Disease Control (CDC). Case-control study of HIV seroconversion in health care workers after percutaneous exposure to HIV-infected blood. *MMWR Morb Mortal Wkly Rep.* 1995;44:929–933.

(b) Prophylactic measures must be instituted and their efficacy evaluated. Various protective procedures, such as gloving and masking, have been devised that, if properly used, appear to be an effective barrier to infection. Institutions must make available necessary barrier materials and insist on their use and other appropriate clinical procedures to inhibit transmission.

(c) Patients may be incorrectly categorized. Toleration of the practice of excluding HIV-positive patients would lead to the exclusion of many persons in serious need of care and the exclusion of many who are incorrectly identified as infected.

(d) The reputation of the profession must be protected. Medical tradition praises those who care for patients at risk to themselves. Medicine's public reputation rests in part on this tradition, and the public expects physicians to act in this way, so far as is reasonable. In the United States, physicians have generally been very responsive and responsible. All major medical organizations have asserted the obligation of physicians to treat patients with HIV infection. The AMA Ethical and Judicial Council states, "A physician may not ethically refuse to treat a patient whose condition is within the physician's realm of competence ... solely because the patient is seropositive for HIV. Persons who are seropositive should not be subjected to discrimination based on fear or prejudice.

Council on Ethical and Judicial Affairs. Code of Medical Ethics of the American Medical Association 2008–2009. 9.131, 334.

4.10.4 Bioterrorism

Bioterrorism refers to the release of toxic or infectious agents among a population, usually in a densly populated area. While the public health and security issues related to bioterrorism are beyond the scope of this book, physicians may be called upon to respond to a bioterrorist attack. Regardless of speciality, physicians should become familiar with the clinical presentation of potential biologic agents, such as pneumonic plague, smallpox, anthrax, and sarin gas. They should also be familiar with the epidemiological methods to distinguish between spontaneous incidence of symptoms and those that might suggest that a clinical case might represent a planned attack. They should also be familiar with reporting methods. It should be noted that a bioterrorism crisis may be of such magnitude and suddenness that many of the usual principles of medical ethics may be challenged.

Also, the moral standing of the health professionals is challenged in such crises. While no physician or nurse has an individual duty to serve, a strong case can be made that health professionals should engage themselves to the extent that they can in meeting the health needs that arise. The public expectation that health professionals freely accept responsibilities toward the health and safety of the population is strong. The general principles of social justice emphasize that those who have certain skills should share them for the public good.

Moreno J. Ethics and bioterrorism. In: Steinbock B, ed. *The Oxford Handbook of Bioethics*. New York, NY: Oxford University Press; 2007:721–734.

4.11 ORGANIZATIONAL ETHICS

Clinical care typically takes place within an organization. Care is given in hospitals or clinics, within health plans, and within the constraints posed by insurers. Clinical decisions and clinical ethics are embedded in these institutional structures and policies.

4.11.1 Question Ten—Are There Conflicts of Interest Within Institutions and Organizations (e.g., Hospitals) That May Affect Clinical Decisions and Patient Welfare?

The answer to this question is clearly "yes." Professionals are often employees of institutions. They are engaged in assuring the safety, stability, and reputation of their institutions. They play a part in formulating policies, overseeing practices, etc. In these many relationships, they may face conflicts of interest. Further, as we have seen earlier, financial viability of institutions may constrain use of resources that patients may need. We do not discuss these specfically, but mention some ways in which conflicts can be resolved or managed in ways that do not adversely impact clinical decisions.

In recent years, the concept of organizational ethics has emerged and has been encouraged by the Joint Commission for Accreditation of Health Care Organizations (JCAHO), which now requires their accredited institutions to develop programs in organizational ethics. *Organizational ethics is the effort on the part of management and staff to express the value assumptions that should guide business or policy decisions within their institutions.* An ethical audit of the institution might reveal the attitudes and opinions of its staff and employees about how well the institution adheres to its stated mission and values. Institutions should have a clear policy and program regarding their mission, range of service, continuous quality improvement in care of patients, guidance on difficult clinical problems, and processes for dispute resolution. There should be institutional mechanisms to formulate, revise, and oversee the implementation of these policies and programs. Organizational ethics should be realized at the highest level of the institution; a high level administrator should be responsible and a committee of the Board of Directors, or equivalent, should be established. Many of the problems noted in preceeding sections of this book can be well managed only within such policies and programs.

Gibson JL, Sibbald R, Connolly E, Singer PA. Organizational ethics. In: Singer PA, Viens AM, eds. *Cambridge Textbook of Bioethics.* Cambridge, MA: Cambridge University Press; 2008:243–250.

Hall R. *An Introduction to Health Care Organizational Ethics*. New York, NY: Oxford University Press; 2000.

4.11.2 Ethics Committees

In the usual practice of medicine, important decisions are made by the patient and physician together. Outside parties do not partake in those decisions unless invited to do so by the principal parties. The growing complexity of the ethical issues in clinical care has stimulated the development of ethics committees and of ethics consultation. At the present time, almost 80% of all US hospitals and 100% of hospitals with more than 300 beds have ethics committees. Ethics committees are advisory groups on policy and on cases that involve ethical issues. It is their responsibility to be familiar with the literature and methods of the field of bioethics and to make available to those who seek their counsel the best informed opinions about issues. Many judicial opinions have endorsed the idea of ethics committees as a means of resolving disputes before the participants are forced to the courts.

Ethics committees differ from institutional review boards (IRBs) which focus on research involving human subjects and function in accordance with federal regulations. Ethics committees deal with policies and problems arising in the care of patients.

Ethics committees develop institutional policies on matters such as DNR or the management of cases of nonbeneficial care. They review problem cases at the request of family or clinicians. Ethics committees may use dispute resolution techniques, such as informal negotiation or mediation, as an alternative to litigation when conflicts arise between patients or families and physicians. It is imperative that patients and families are informed of the existence and functions of the ethics committee. Although the number of ethics committees has increased greatly in recent years, and very few US hospitals are without one, there are no rigorous studies to evaluate the effectiveness of these committees. Relatively few committee members or consultants have advanced training in clinical ethics. Nevertheless, it is generally agreed that an effective ethics committee should have the following features:

(a) Endorsement and support from the hospital administration and the medical and nursing staff. That support should include sufficient resources for the committee to function efficiently. The committee should be located clearly and appropriately in the institution's organizational chart, with designated lines of reporting.

(b) Members should be persons who are respected by their peers. The committee should also have members from outside the health care organization who represent a nonprofessional view of problems and may be able to speak for certain communities served by the organization. Members should meet regularly and keep records of their deliberations and of case consultations. Records should be maintained as confidential, according to the relevant laws.

(c) The committee should establish methods of informing the staff of its existence and role and the procedures whereby it is contacted. Educational functions, such as occasional grand rounds or noon conferences, should be sponsored.

(d) Members and potential members should be given the opportunity and support to pursue education in medical ethics. Many educational opportunities are now available throughout the country.

Lo B. Ethics committees and case consultation. In: Lo B, ed. *Resolving Ethical Dilemmas. A Guide for Clinicians*. 3rd ed. Philadelphia, PA: Lippincott Williams and Wilkins; 2005:111–116.

Post LF, Blustein J, Dubler NN. *Handbook for Health Care Ethics Committees*. Baltimore, MD: The Johns Hopkins University Press; 2007.

4.11.3 Ethics Consultation

Many hospitals and other health care institutions have employed ethics consultants or have authorized members of the ethics committee to engage in consultations on ethical problems arising in particular cases. Ethics consultation is modeled on the familiar practice of professional consultation. Certain persons with particular knowledge and experience are available to clinicians and patients, to review the facts of a particular case and offer informed and prudent counsel suited to the case. There are now persons with graduate training in bioethics and with mentored training in clinical ethics consultation. An increasing number of large hospitals retain the services of such persons. They should be given appropriate hospital accreditation. Such persons can be of invaluable service to clinicians in dealing with complex cases. The conclusions of ethics committees and of ethics consultants are advisory only and usually reported to the attending physician.

The central goal of ethics consultation is to improve the process and outcome of care by identifying, analyzing, and working to resolve ethical problems encountered in individual cases, such as the ones described in this book. To achieve this goal, it is necessary to identify the issue that precipitated the consultation and to facilitate resolution through patient and staff education and the opportunity for informed and respectful discussion of the problem. Consultation may also help deeply involved parties see cases in a perspective different than their own.

Competency for ethics consultation includes knowledge of bioethics, the relevant professional codes of ethics, and relevant health law. An ethics consultant should also have sufficient knowledge of medicine to understand the clinical situation and converse with clinicians about it, demonstrate skill at moral reasoning, and have the ability to build moral consensus in a group. A number of educational programs offer degrees and certificates in bioethics. Ethics consultation has been evaluated in several retrospective studies that showed a significantly high level of patient and physician satisfaction with the consultation. Several small studies suggest that ethics consultation does not increase mortality and does decrease length of stay in intensive care units. Standards for ethics consultation have been developed by the American Society for Bioethics and Humanities, the leading professional organzation for bioethicists.

American Society of Bioethics and Humanities. *Core Competencies for Health Care Ethics Consultation*, 1998.
Aulisio MP, Arnold RM, Youngner S. *Ethics Consultation: From Theory to Practice*. Baltimore, MD: The Johns Hopkins Press; 2003.

RECOMMENDATION. We recommend that ethics committees and ethics consultants employ the method of analysis presented in this book.

4P PEDIATRIC NOTES

4.1P Organ Transplantation for Children

Successful organ transplantation depends on having donors that are HLA-compatible. Such donors are often siblings. One may ask, is it ethical to take a kidney or bone marrow from a healthy child for a seriously ill sibling? An ethical response must assume that the child would willingly donate, if able to do so. However, in formulating an answer to this "substituted judgment or implicit consent," the major question concerns the risk to which a healthy child is put for the possible benefit of his or her sibling. In our view, it is indefensible to impose the significant risks of removal of a kidney without consent; it is defensible to suggest the notably lesser risks of donation of bone marrow. Needless to say, the negotiations with family and with the child require the utmost delicacy, the psychologic implications for the children in the event of either failure or success must be recognized, and the legal requirements in the jurisdiction must be complied with. Should there be parental disagreement, the plan should be abandoned.

Frankel LR, Goldworth A, Rorty MV, Silverman WA, eds. *Ethical Dilemmas in Pediatrics. Cases and Commentaries* [Part III]. Cambridge, MA: Cambridge University Press; 2005:157–220.

Locator

This locator gives in bold type the Section number in which the item is discussed, followed by the page numbers. **P** designates Pediatric Note.

The Four Topics Chart

Medical Indications

The Principles of Beneficence and Nonmaleficence

1. What is the patient's medical problem? Is the problem acute? chronic? critical? reversible? emergent? terminal?
2. What are the goals of treatment?
3. In what circumstances are medical treatments not indicated?
4. What are the probabilities of success of various treatment options?
5. In sum, how can this patient be benefited by medical and nursing care, and how can harm be avoided?

Patient References

The Principle of Respect for Autonomy

1. Has the patient been informed of benefits and risks, understood this information, and given consent?
2. Is the patient mentally capable and legally competent, and is there evidence of incapacity?
3. If mentally capable, what preferences about treatment is the patient stating?
4. If incapacitated, has the patient expressed prior preferences?
5. Who is the appropriate surrogate to make decisions for the incapacitated patient?
6. Is the patient unwilling or unable to cooperate with medical treatment? If so, why?

Quality of Life

The Principles of Beneficence and Nonmaleficence and Respect for Autonomy

1. What are the prospects, with or without treatment, for a return to normal life, and what physical, mental, and social deficits might the patient experience even if treatment succeeds?
2. On what grounds can anyone judge that some quality of life would be undesirable for a patient who cannot make or express such a judgment?
3. Are there biases that might prejudice the provider's evaluation of the patient's quality of life?
4. What ethical issues arise concerning improving or enhancing a patient's quality of life?
5. Do quality-of-life assessments raise any questions regarding changes in treatment plans, such as forgoing life-sustaining treatment?
6. What are plans and rationale to forgo life-sustaining treatment?
7. What is the legal and ethical status of suicide?

Contextual Features

The Principles of Justice and Fairness

1. Are there professional, interprofessional, or business interests that might create conflicts of interest in the clinical treatment of patients?
2. Are there parties other than clinicians and patients, such as family members, who have an interest in clinical decisions?
3. What are the limits imposed on patient confidentiality by the legitimate interests of third parties?
4. Are there financial factors that create conflicts of interest in clinical decisions?
5. Are there problems of allocation of scarce health resources that might affect clinical decisions?
6. Are there religious issues that might influence clinical decisions?
7. What are the legal issues that might affect clinical decisions?
8. Are there considerations of clinical research and education that might affect clinical decisions?
9. Are there issues of public health and safety that affect clinical decisions?
10. Are there conflicts of interest within institutions and organizations (e.g., hospitals) that may affect clinical decisions and patient welfare?

Jonsen AR, Siegler M, Winslade WJ. *Clinical Ethics: A Practical Approach to Ethical Decisions in Clinical Medicine.* 7th ed. New York, NY: McGraw-Hill; 2010.